Advanced Praise

T0372806

This is one of those rare books, clearly meticulously researched and written, that we have needed for many years; one that I genuinely feel will change the well-being landscape for everyone involved in dance. Monika draws on a huge depth of personal and professional experience which is clearly evident throughout this truly remarkable book, and my hope is that every teacher and teacher-in-training worldwide gets their hands on it.

> Fiona Sutherland, *MSc (Nut & Diet), RYT,*
> *Nutrition Consultant, The Australian*
> *Ballet School*

Nourishing Dance is a true gem challenging diet culture and offering a comprehensive guide for dancers, and those working with dancers, to stay informed on best practices for supportive care. Monika brings together science, research, and personal experience from her dietitian and dancer perspectives, creating an invaluable body of work and impactful call to action.

> Josh Spell, *LICSW, Consulting mental*
> *health therapist at Pacific Northwest Ballet*

Comprehensive in scope and grounded by scientific research, this indispensable book will serve as a resource for parents and for all those invested in the health and well-being of dancers. It should be required reading for dance teachers, administrators, and artistic directors, as well as for every health professional who cares for dancers.

> David S. Weiss, *MD, FAAOS, Performing arts*
> *medicine specialist, Orthopedic consultant*
> *to numerous NYC dance companies and*
> *Broadway theatrical productions*

Nourishing Dance is a comprehensive guide and a must-read for dance educators, parents, staff, choreographers, and anyone responsible for developing dancers. Monika Saigal demonstrates the importance of education and the use of language as she challenges common practices in the dance industry in the name of "tradition." She provides extensive support for the prevention of eating disorders and provides essential information on nutrition for dancers.

> Blanca Huertas-Agnew, *MFA, Dance*
> *Program Director and Assistant Teaching*
> *Professor at Drexel University*

Monika reminds us that dancer health can only be meaningfully improved to the extent that the prevailing dance culture improves too. This book provides clear guidance not only for dancers but also for those shaping the culture to better support them. Directors, teachers, choreographers, parents, health profession-als—read these words and put them into action!

Philippa Ziegenhardt, *MACA, Counsellor,*
Stageminded.com and former School
Counsellor at The Australian Ballet School

Monika Saigal's meticulously researched and essential work *is* nourishment for the dance field and for the humans who dedicate their hearts, minds, and bodies to its work.

Elizabeth Gillaspy, *Professor, TCU School*
for Classical & Contemporary Dance

Nourishing Dance is a nutrient-dense resource that expertly highlights the defi-ciency of nutrition-based education, the sociocultural influences on body image and the risk of developing eating disorders in the dance community. A must read for anyone who employs, trains and cares for dancers.

Andrea Zujko, *PT, DPT, OCS, COMT,*
Clinic Manager, Westside Dance Physical
Therapy, Adjunct Faculty, NYU Tisch
School of the Arts, Founder, Dance
Medicine Education Initiative

In *Nourishing Dance* Monika Saigal has deftly blended her experience as a dancer with the expertise she has gained in her subsequent career devoted to the health and well-being of dancers. The result is a rich, essential resource for parents, teachers, coaches, and choreographers who support or come in contact with dancers at any level. I recommend it enthusiastically!

Mary Margaret Holt, *Dean, University of*
Oklahoma College of Fine Arts, former
Director of the OU School of Dance,
choreographer, and former professional
dancer

Advising dancers is difficult if you haven't been in their shoes, but Monika Saigal has this box checked: her dual expertise in dance and nutrition practically jumps off the page. The information she shares is so important for not only dancers to have, but everyone in a dancer's orbit. I appreciate how she addresses disordered eating in a way that feels both practically useful and honest, and also absent of hyperbole. I wish I had this resource when I was a professional dancer!

Sasha Gorrell, *PhD, Assistant Professor,*
Eating Disorders Program, University
of California, San Francisco, Licensed
Clinical Psychologist, and former
professional ballet dancer

Monika Saigal's *Nourishing Dance* is the ultimate book for education on and prevention of eating disorders and disordered eating in the dance community. The breadth and depth of the topics covered in this book—how to recognize and prevent disordered thoughts and behaviors, what language to use to communicate skillfully, reality-checking nutrition information to support dancers' athleticism—will make it a resource you return to again and again. Whether you are a dancer, teacher, dietitian, parent, or director of a dance program, you will transform your knowledge of diet, eating, body image, and how to support the dancers in your life.

> **Jenna Hollenstein**, *MS, RD, CDN, author
> of* Eat to Love: A Mindful Guide to
> Transform Your Relationship with Food,
> Body, and Life *and* Intuitive Eating for
> Life: How Mindfulness Can Deepen and
> Sustain Your Intuitive Eating Practice

Monika Saigal's book *Nourishing Dance* addresses the difficult subject of how some of the current practices in dance training can negatively affect the health of dancers. It is a comprehensive and thoughtful guide to the problems that can arise around body image, misinformation about food and nutrition, and negative aspects of diet culture in the dance world and in general. The book provides clear nutritional guidelines and concrete steps to address some of the detrimental psychological pitfalls of the dance community's entrenched customs and traditions. I hope all dancers, dance teachers, artistic staff, and dance medicine practitioners read this book and use it as a valuable guide.

> **Julie Daugherty**, *Company Physical
> Therapist, American Ballet Theatre*

Nourishing Dance

Nourishing Dance: An Essential Guide on Nutrition, Body Image, and Eating Disorders is written with an insider's understanding of the unique needs and pressures of the dance world and the expertise of an eating disorder specialist, dietitian, clinician, and educator. This much-needed resource provides research-based, practical approaches to help dancers fuel optimally, nourish a peaceful relationship with food, and nurture more positive and resilient body image.

Under-fueling, body dissatisfaction, eating disorders, and disordered eating are far too common among dancers. Despite the prevalence of these issues in dancers across genres, and their negative impacts on dancers' physical and mental health and performance, they have not been adequately addressed in the dance community. Improving dancers' health and well-being is necessary for both dancers and the art form to thrive, and everyone involved in the training and care of dancers can play an important role in this mission.

Nourishing Dance provides essential information on nutrition, body image, and eating disorder prevention to help parents, teachers, staff, choreographers, leadership, athletic trainers, coaches, and healthcare professionals contribute to making the dance world a healthier and safer place for dancers.

Monika Saigal, MS, RD, CEDS, CDN, is a Registered Dietitian Nutritionist, Certified Eating Disorders Specialist, and former professional dancer specializing in nutrition for dancers and the prevention and treatment of eating disorders/disordered eating. Monika has over 15 years of experience providing nutrition counseling to dancers and performing artists in her private practice and extensive experience working with dance organizations—from small studios to world-renowned schools, conservatories, and companies. Monika regularly delivers workshops for dancers as well as specialized trainings for dance educators, staff, parents, and healthcare professionals.

Nourishing Dance

An Essential Guide on Nutrition,
Body Image, and Eating Disorders

Monika Saigal

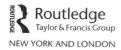
Routledge
Taylor & Francis Group

NEW YORK AND LONDON

Designed cover image: Ivana Mundja

First published 2024
by Routledge
605 Third Avenue, New York, NY 10158

and by Routledge
4 Park Square, Milton Park, Abingdon, Oxon, OX14 4RN

Routledge is an imprint of the Taylor & Francis Group, an informa business

© 2024 Monika Saigal

ISBN: 978-1-032-43212-0 (hbk)
ISBN: 978-1-032-43211-3 (pbk)
ISBN: 978-1-003-36617-1 (ebk)

DOI: 10.4324/9781003366171

Typeset in Sabon
by Deanta Global Publishing Services, Chennai, India

For my Papito—generosity, strength, and resilience personified.

Disclaimer

The information provided in this book is for educational purposes only. The content of this book is not intended to diagnose, treat, cure, or prevent any condition or disease. This book is not intended to be and should not be used as a substitute for professional care or advice, clinical or otherwise. This book does not create any provider/patient or author/client relationship. You should seek the advice of a qualified and licensed healthcare professional for any questions or concerns about your health or the health of a dancer in your life. The author specifically disclaims any liability, loss, or risk that is incurred as a direct or indirect consequence of the use and application of any contents of this book.

Contents

xii *Contents*

xii *Contents*

Figures

Tables

Note to the Reader on Language Choices

As a first-generation American with parents from India and Argentina, I understand the importance of recognizing how each person's unique background and culture shapes their identity and impacts the experiences they have and the challenges they face. Unfortunately, word count constraints require me to be reductive at times. For the sake of conciseness, I have chosen to use the term "dancers of color" in some places to describe dancers from minoritized/marginalized groups (e.g., Black, Hispanic, Latinx, Native American, Asian, South Asian, Pacific Islander, and more). The use of this term is not meant to convey the idea that dancers of color are part of a monolithic group or to minimize the differences among these diverse identities and cultures.

Regarding sex and gender, I have chosen to use they/them pronouns instead of he/him/she/her. The terms "male"/"female" and related terms (e.g., "men"/"women") are used to correspond with the language used in the referenced literature (most of the resources cited in this book use the male/female binary). The use of this terminology is not meant to imply that male and female are the only two sexes or boy/man and girl/woman are the only two genders. Although research is lacking on intersex and non-binary dancers, I have attempted to present information in this book that has applicability to all dancers.

When weight descriptions such as "normal weight" and "overweight" are used (e.g., to correspond with cited literature), the terms are presented in quotation marks because these classifications are based on the problematic body mass index (BMI) (or other equally controversial weight-for-height calculations/categories). In addition, quotation marks are used to acknowledge that terms such as "overweight," "obese," and "obesity" are stigmatizing and harmful compared to more neutral descriptors of body size such as "in a larger body" or "higher weight individual."

Finally, the idea of what's healthy has become warped in our society. The word is often used to describe attitudes, behaviors, and outcomes that have less to do with health and well-being, and more to do with control of one's shape, size, or appearance (e.g., restrictive and compensatory approaches to eating, punishing exercise). Yet, for conciseness—and because we don't really have a good alternative word—I use the term "healthy" throughout this book. When I use this word, I am referring to eating (or exercising) in a way that supports physical and mental health and that is enjoyable, flexible, and adaptive. A healthy mindset is one that prioritizes caring for the body and supports a peaceful relationship with food and your body. Health promotion has to account for individual needs, circumstances, and preferences. So, when I use the word "healthy," I recognize that it means something different for everyone. What's healthy for a dancer (and each of us) also changes based on our stage in life and multiple other factors.

Prologue

Everything Is Beautiful at the Ballet?

The lights. The costumes. The scenery. The dancers embodying the music and painting magnificent pictures with their bodies. My desire to dance was sparked by my first time attending a ballet performance. I was in awe, moved, and inspired. Over time and the more I immersed myself in dance, the more my love and appreciation for the art form grew.

On a personal level, dance gifted me with an important vehicle of expression and an escape from life's hardships, though being a part of the dance world wasn't without its difficulties. Like many dancers, I thought of the barre as my home and those I shared the studio with became family. As with any family, there may be problems and dysfunction that aren't visible to those on the outside or even to some on the inside. Family members who do recognize a problem may ignore it because they don't know what to do or fear the repercussions of disrupting the system. So, we present a picture to the world that is a well-rehearsed performance. Everything is beautiful at the ballet ... at least from the view in front of the curtain.

Looking Behind the Curtain

Our teacher lined us up in front of the mirror after class. With disgust displayed across his face and in his voice, he said "Turn around and look at yourselves. You better just eat lettuce leaves between now and the performances."

The choreographer admonished the dancers after his rehearsal: "You are not in shape for this piece—especially a few of you. Time to cut out sugar. You should just be eating chicken and vegetables to get ready for the show."

The first statement was directed at me and my teen and pre-teen dancer peers at the end of ballet class in my hometown studio in New Orleans in 1990. The second was said to my client, an adult professional dancer, at the end of rehearsal with a modern dance company in Europe in 2020. These two troubling experiences are so similar despite being separated by decades, continents, and dance genres. How can we still be in a place where body shaming and harmful nutrition advice are so commonplace and accepted in the dance world?

Did my teacher and my client's choreographer intend to harm us? Did they understand the impact their words would have, especially given the power and gender dynamics in the room? Probably not. Although there are undoubtedly and tragically those in the dance world who knowingly hurt and abuse dancers, I don't believe they are representative of the vast majority of teachers, directors, and choreographers. And yet, harm is done and done quite often. Dance training involves traditions passed down from generation to generation. Unfortunately, traditions like body shaming, encouraging starvation, and (sometimes public) weigh-ins are passed down as well without asking the question, "This was done to me, but is it what's best for my dancers?" So, the cycle of pain continues.

Lessons That Last a Lifetime

I wish the stories I shared were the worst things I and my dancer friends experienced through the years, or that I hear so often now from my dancer clients. It doesn't matter if a trusted dance professional makes these comments with the misguided intention of motivating, inspiring, or helping a dancer reach their full potential. Impact matters more than intention. As you'll see illustrated in this book, or perhaps have experienced yourself, the effects of body shaming and practices that encourage disordered eating are enduring.

The critique about a part of a dancer's body that is "too big."

Food policing framed as helping a dancer take care of their body.

The pathologizing of normal body changes.

These messages teach dancers how to think and feel about their body and how to nourish and care for themselves. Whether subtle or overt, repeated messages or a singular statement, the impacts of these lessons can last a lifetime.

The Pursuit of Perfection

Body image dissatisfaction, eating disorders, disordered eating, and underfueling are common among dancers—a harsh reality confirmed by research that is not surprising to most of us who have spent any time involved in the dance world. Dance is an aesthetic art form which, depending on genre, may prefer and accept only a narrow range of "ideal" body types. As aesthetic athletes, dancers are faced with a unique challenge of needing significant strength and energy to meet the physical demands of training and performing, while also often being required to conform to the strict visual expectations of their art.

Dance is highly competitive and, even for the most talented dancers, requires discipline, dedication, and sacrifice as well as a persistent drive to achieve the unachievable: perfection. The pressures dancers face are intense and yet for most, their training does not provide them with the knowledge, tools, or support they need to remain healthy in this challenging environment. Dance teachers and staff face a difficult dilemma as well. They are expected to push dancers to reach their full potential, to do everything possible to help them achieve their dreams, and to train them to be prepared for the realities and expectations of the dance world. But teachers aren't given the training or support to do this in a way that protects dancers from harmful messages and influences. Many teachers and staff know something needs to change but don't know how to be a part of the change they wish to see.

In the U.S. alone, there are millions of dance students in studios and college dance programs. Dance training, even for those who don't wish or intend to pursue it professionally, can significantly influence a dancer's eating habits, sense of self-worth, and body image. A minuscule number of dance students actually go on to dance professionally—some may become teachers or choreographers, but the majority of dance students will not remain in the field in any professional capacity. They may however become audience members, potential donors, and future parents of dance students. How will their personal experiences in the dance world shape their future involvement in the art?

When dancers connect their poor body image, low self-esteem, and/or disordered eating habits to their experiences in dance, the impacts can be far reaching and of significant consequence. Many of my former dancer clients who feel scarred by their own experiences, especially with body shaming, don't want their children to dance. Or they might say, "Maybe hip-hop or tap. But no ballet." They are trying to protect their children from the harmful messages and practices they were exposed to. Some former dancers decide they no longer want to attend dance performances. Others need to take a long break to heal before they can see a dance performance without reliving the pain of their former lives. We also need to consider what happens when dancers who have not yet recovered from an eating disorder or their own body hatred become teachers or choreographers or take on positions of leadership. How does their own relationship with food and their body inform their interactions and work with dancers? The dance world can no longer afford to focus solely on the end without evaluating the impact of the means.

Although eating disorders, disordered eating, and inadequate fueling are prevalent in dance, and despite the fact that these conditions can have devastating effects on a dancer's performance, career, and physical and mental health, these issues aren't discussed enough and certainly have not been adequately addressed. One of the reasons I wrote this book is to bring these areas of dancer health into the foreground: how can we tackle the problem if we aren't talking about it?

The Missing Element in Dance Training

Dance is one of my true loves and being a dancer remains an integral part of my identity—once a dancer, always a dancer. Dance has given me countless gifts including cherished memories and friendships and an outlet that still fuels my soul. Although my professional dance career was cut much too short by multiple injuries with difficult, protracted recoveries, and even though I've had to do my own work to heal physically and emotionally from some of the negative aspects of dance, I am immensely grateful for my life as a dancer. And without my dance story, I wouldn't have my current career.

For all I learned in my dance training, there were glaring gaps as well. I was not taught about nutrition or how to properly care for my body, neither during my years as a student nor in my time as a professional. I did receive a lot of advice and tips on dieting and weight loss from friends, family, and teachers, but I never learned how to eat in a way that could help improve my performance or prevent injury. I did not know how to nourish myself in a way that supported my physical and mental health. No one talked about eating disorders—but eating disorders, disordered eating, harmful weight control practices, and body bashing were all around me and seemed like a normal and accepted part of being a dancer.

What I experienced and witnessed led me to pursue a career as a dietitian specializing in nutrition for dancers and the prevention and treatment of eating disorders. The past 15 plus years I've spent as a dance dietitian working with dancers and dance organizations have highlighted some important things. The problems that the dance world needs to urgently address are widespread and not isolated to any one city or country or continent. A lot has changed since the time I was a dancer (e.g., the advent of foam rollers and understanding the importance of cross-training), but unfortunately many of the areas that need to change (e.g., body shaming, disordered eating, harmful nutrition advice, and lack of diversity) haven't changed enough or at all.

I strongly believe that nutrition education, including a focus on nourishing both physical and mental health, needs to be included as an ongoing part of dance training. I hope that teaching dancers how to properly care for their mind and body will one day be the standard—one essential tool in the arsenal we will need to make the dance world a healthier and safer place. And for those who feel that devoting time and resources to these areas of dancer health will detract from training, I say the opposite is true: when dancers have the knowledge and support they need to practice good self-care, it improves their dancing and benefits the dance world as a whole.

For the Love of Dance

I love working with dancers. I love how our experiences from this unique world connect us. I love being a part of helping dancers heal from punishing eating habits and critical self-talk to find their way to a healthy and peaceful relationship with food and their body. I love seeing their love of dance restored and watching them thrive as a dancer and human connected to their authentic self. But the more time I've spent working with dancers, the more I've realized that a dancer's ability to develop healthy habits and a healthy mindset is significantly limited by an unsupportive environment.

When I speak with dance teachers, staff, parents, and healthcare professionals about eating disorder prevention, or present at dance medicine and eating disorder conferences, or collaborate with other colleagues who work in dance, I hear related sentiments. Dancers say it's difficult to make changes without support from teachers and leadership. Parents and healthcare providers say they can't help their dancers make positive changes when the schools and companies encourage the opposite. Teachers and staff say they need buy-in from leadership. Artistic leadership say they believe change is needed, but they can't disregard what is currently expected in the dance world. Everyone is right. If we want to improve the health and well-being of dancers, it will take all of us.

I think many dancers would agree that the dance environment has a negative, or at best neutral, influence on their eating habits, relationship with food, and body image. Wouldn't it be wonderful if the dance world was instead a place that could be a positive force in these critical areas of a dancer's (and human's) development? I believe it can be. It needs to be if we want the art form we all love so much to not just survive and stay relevant but to continue to move and inspire.

Knowing Better, Doing Better

The poster on the ceiling of my childhood bedroom was a picture of a ballet dancer in a gauzy cream-colored costume with the quote, "If you can imagine it, you can achieve it. If you can dream it, you can become it." If we can imagine a dance world that trains dancers in a way that helps (rather than harms) their physical and mental health, we can achieve it. But we need to be willing to do the hard work of compassionately exploring, unlearning, relearning, and growing.

Dance teachers are experts on helping dancers improve technique and artistry, but what if they all knew how to speak about the body in a way that helps dancers develop positive body image? Parents do everything they can to nurture and protect their children, but what if they all knew how to insulate their dancers from the harms of diet culture and help them nourish their bodies in a way that supports their physical and mental health? Dance medicine providers dedicate their lives to caring for dancers, but what if their practices consistently reinforced messages that enhanced the health of the whole dancer? Leadership wants dancers who support their vision for their company, but what if the mission of the company indisputably supported the dancers' health and longevity?

We cannot do better until we know better. I want everyone involved in the training and care of dancers—parents, teachers, staff, choreographers, leadership, other dance providers (Pilates teachers, athletic trainers, strength and conditioning coaches), and healthcare professionals (physicians, psychotherapists, physical and occupational therapists, dietitians)—to have the necessary knowledge and tools to be part of the change that is so needed in the dance world. We each have a critical role to play so that dance training can be synonymous with helping dancers to be healthy mentally and physically.

Self-Compassion Is Key

Before we begin our journey together, a note on self-compassion. I believe that each of you wants the best for dancers and the fact that you are reading this book confirms it. Exploring the areas that need to change in the dance world is not about placing blame; it is about each one of us taking responsibility for our part in doing better. When we care so much about the dancers and clients we work with, it can be painful when we realize the potential harm we may have caused to others. But we are all humans in a never-ending process of growing and learning, which makes mistakes inevitable and inadvertent harm probable.

As you read this book, you may begin to consider things that you wish to have said or done differently. When this happens, I encourage you to try to be compassionate with yourself rather than harsh or judgmental. Self-compassion means being kind and understanding to ourselves when we're hurting or when we feel like we've failed or feel like we aren't good enough. It is an invaluable skill for us to cultivate within ourselves and to nurture in dancers.

What to Expect from This Book

Nourishing Dance is the first book of this kind, offering a unique perspective based on my experience as a dancer, eating disorder specialist, dietitian, clinician, and educator. Guidelines and recommendations are based on scientific research and developed with an understanding of the unique needs and pressures of the dance world. Case studies are interspersed throughout the book to enhance learning (names and identifying details have been changed to protect confidentiality and some of the cases are an amalgamation of several different dancers). Each chapter ends with a summary of take-home "Main Pointes" and "Notes," which much like notes given at the end of a rehearsal or performance, offer prompts for personal reflection to help you identify areas that may benefit from exploration or perhaps need some healing.

This book provides essential information on nutrition, body image, and eating disorders that will benefit anyone involved in the training and care of dancers and is relevant for dancers of all levels and genres. However, practical applications will vary depending on your role (e.g., teacher vs. parent vs. healthcare professional). Act I sets the stage with an exploration of diet culture, how its messages (and harms) get amplified in the dance world, and how dieting, misinformation, disordered eating, and other factors contribute to under-fueling in dancers. This section concludes with an in-depth discussion of eating disorders in dancers, including prevalence, risk factors, warning signs/symptoms, and what to do and not do if you suspect a dancer may have disordered eating or an eating disorder.

Without proper detection and intervention, inadequate fueling, eating disorders, and disordered eating can have dire consequences. Fortunately, these serious conditions are preventable and treatable. Act II focuses on various aspects of prevention including a discussion on the importance of language. I cover how to speak about food, weight, and bodies in a way that helps (rather than harms) and provide guidance on how to shift language and messaging to create a protective environment that cultivates healthy habits and a healthy mindset in dancers.

Act III covers nutrition, injury, body image, and self-care topics to help nourish the whole dancer. I interviewed dancers as well as physical therapists and psychotherapists who specialize in working with dancers for this book, and this section shares their experiences and recommendations. When you complete this book, you will have a greater understanding of the pressures and issues dancers face that compromise their mental and physical health. I hope you will come away with knowledge, ideas, and inspiration to be a part of the way forward. Thank you for being here. I'm excited to begin our journey toward improving the health and well-being of dancers.

Act I

Setting the Stage

1 Dancing in Diet Culture

I integrated "the mind set": a dancer must diet, she must be hungry. This was one of the ways to become a dancer. If I hadn't had all these preconceived ideas, if I had not assimilated them, I am sure that I would not have been on so many diets.
~Belinda,* female professional ballet dancer[1]

Have you ever felt the desire to lose weight to improve your appearance? To change your size or shape to feel better in some way? Felt pressure to lose weight to improve your health? Have you ever felt proud of yourself for eating the "right" foods or chastised yourself for indulging in the "wrong" foods? Have you ever celebrated the number on the scale or size on the clothing tag getting smaller? Felt shame if either of those numbers increased? Felt disappointment if your shape or musculature didn't change as you hoped for?

These are the influences of diet culture. Messages so ubiquitous and widely accepted that many of us haven't stopped to question their origin, validity, or impact. This chapter will cover diet culture both independent of the dance world and within it.

What Is Diet Culture?

Diet culture is a system of socially conditioned beliefs that tells us:

1. Thinner bodies and certain body types defined by some "ideal" musculature or shape are better bodies—healthier, more attractive, more desirable, more successful, more virtuous.
2. We can achieve the "ideal" body by changing and closely regulating our eating and exercise habits.
3. There is a "right" and "wrong" way to eat defined by consuming "good" food and reducing or eliminating "bad" foods.
4. Controlling our eating and managing our weight are evidence of moral superiority.

DOI: 10.4324/9781003366171-2

Diet culture has been exerting its influence for far longer than any of us have been around. The association between controlling what and how much we eat as a means of achieving health and beauty can be traced back to the ancient Greeks.[2] Centuries ago, religions began linking food restraint and deprivation with morality and salvation,[3] laying the groundwork for categorizing foods as good or bad and viewing eating habits as right or wrong. The medical community has been instrumental in associating weight with health, though at one time, the messaging was the opposite of what we hear today (i.e., heavier bodies were preferred). Throughout history, in addition to religion and medicine, art, literature, politics, business interests, fashion, and the media have all played a part in shaping and perpetuating the messages of diet culture that we are now bombarded with.

Thinness has not always been synonymous with health or beauty. Full-figured, fleshier female bodies were the favored aesthetic during the Renaissance. You may be familiar with some of the 17th-century paintings by artist Peter Paul Rubens who celebrated the plump, curvy female form.[3] However, not all larger bodies were deemed acceptable—even in Rubens's time, they had to have the "correct" proportions.[3]

At the end of the 19th century, low (not high) body weight was considered a health issue. American doctors discouraged thinness, and life insurance companies denied policies to "underweight" individuals due to the prevailing belief that higher-weight bodies were better equipped to fight infectious diseases.[4] Although a slender physique was becoming more fashionable, the culture of thinness was considered an epidemic which was not only unhealthy but also a threat to the nation.[3]

For much of history, larger bodies were seen as a sign of prosperity and health whereas thin bodies were a sign of poverty and illness.[5] While there are still a few cultures and societies in which larger bodies are seen as healthier and more desirable, these views seem to be shifting with increased exposure to Western ideals.[5-7] Nevertheless, the overwhelming message perpetuated by modern-day diet culture is that thinner/leaner is better.

When studying the history of diet culture† you'll find a system where what's old is made new again and again. Many of the same weight-loss methods promoted ages ago are still present today: low carb diets, calorie counting, fasting, food combining, diet pills, and obsessive weighing and measuring of food and the body. Even when diet claims lack evidence regarding their long-term efficacy, have been disproven, or have been found to be harmful, they remain—continuously recycled and repurposed for over 150 years.

Looking back at some of the weight-loss methods promoted in the past (e.g., diet pills with arsenic, tapeworms, and cold baths!),[5,8] you might question how anyone would think those methods were a good idea. But much like today, dieters throughout history have been influenced by medical experts, celebrity endorsements, and popular opinion. If a doctor recommends an intervention, we assume it's safe—the history of prescribing fen-phen‡ for weight loss is just one example of how harmful this assumption can be. If a celebrity we admire says "this diet plan worked for me," we believe we can achieve the same results, even if the celebrity's results are primarily due to plastic surgery. And when our friends, family, and the media send the message that "x" diet is the way to go, we become convinced that we should follow it too.

Diet culture is a powerful force that makes us believe we are not good enough as we are. Diet culture tells us our value and acceptance are based on how close we are to meeting the body type that has been deemed ideal. But this "ideal" is constantly shifting and never quite attainable. Be thin, but not too thin. Be strong, but not too muscular or bulky. Curves are out. Curves are in, but only in the right proportions. Diet culture convinces us that an inability to attain the "ideal" body and the rights and privileges that come with it is our fault, making us vulnerable to the false promises of diet after diet. The influence of diet culture is so strong that we are willing to try just about anything to change our body, regardless of the impact on our well-being, and even when the methods are hard to reconcile with science or common sense.

Diet Culture Is Everywhere

Most of us have been raised in diet culture; its messages and influence surround us. When we are immersed in something and it is so embedded in our way of life, we may not notice it or see its impact on us. There is also a camaraderie and bonding aspect to diet culture that adds pressure to participate and makes it difficult to reject for fear of not fitting in, isolation, or missing out. Only when we become aware of the presence and effects of diet culture can we begin working to undo its harm. Table 1.1 lists some of the ways diet culture may show up in your life.

Diet culture can significantly shape how we think and feel. For example, here are some things you may believe because of diet culture's influence:

• If a diet isn't working, the person following the diet needs more discipline and willpower.
• Being in a larger body is the result of "overeating" and/or eating "bad" foods.
• A thinner/leaner body is a healthier body.
• If a person in a larger body has health issues, they are at fault because they chose not to take care of themselves properly.
• Certain foods are allowed only if you earn them (e.g., with exercise or by being "good").
• Tricking your body into eating less and not responding to hunger are accomplishments.
• Losing weight will make you feel better, look better, and help you live the life you've always dreamed of.

- You should wait until you achieve your ideal body before you do things you want to do (e.g., date, go on a vacation, buy new clothes, pursue a job opportunity).

In recent years, "diet" has become more of a dirty word, but that hasn't slowed the influence of shape-shifting diet culture. With increased attention to the fact that diets don't work (discussed in more detail shortly), the diet industry has rebranded its messaging to promote "lifestyle" changes and "wellness" plans and a supposed focus on body positivity. The explicit messages of diet culture have shifted somewhat, but the implicit messages haven't changed much at all, nor have the methods. We're sold products and plans that say they are about being strong and healthy, not about being skinny. But the images of health and strength used to exemplify what to aspire to are almost exclusively of thin bodies that also typify Eurocentric beauty standards. And even though the sneaky diet industry tells us these new plans aren't diets, the methods are still based on restrictive, rigid, and compensatory approaches to eating and exercise. Despite the purported focus on health and wellness, these new "not-a-diet" diets usually lead to the opposite—harming our physical and mental health as we strive for the unattainable.

Feeling bad about ourselves and blaming our bodies sends us on an endless quest to change our size and shape to try to feel better. But, as illustrated in Figure 1.1, those are rarely the outcomes of dieting. Is diet culture benefiting us or just continuing to create huge profits for the multibillion-dollar (and growing) diet industry?

Table 1.1 How You May Encounter Diet Culture

Family members, friends, peers, public figures, and influencers discussing the latest diet that they are following
People boasting about how they haven't eaten all day
Food and ingredients categorized in dichotomous ways such as good/bad, healthy/unhealthy, clean/toxic, real/fake
Rules for what/when/how much to eat and other practices that should be followed (e.g., chew each bite X number of times)
Complimenting and celebrating weight loss and smaller bodies
People saying "I feel fat" to describe negative feelings (vs. saying they feel "skinny" when they feel good)
Jokes and insults that link fatness with undesirable qualities (e.g., laziness)
Getting or giving unsolicited diet or weight-loss advice
Framing exercise in terms of burning off or making up for "indulgences"
Advertisements and product placements in movies, on television, and on social media for weight-loss/metabolism-boosting supplements, diet foods, diet plans, exercise equipment, etc.

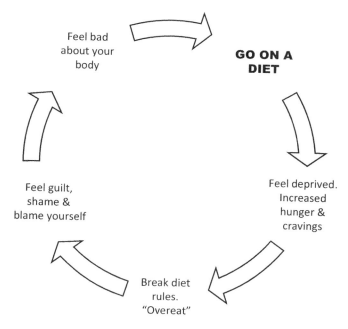

Figure 1.1 The Dieting Cycle. Note: "Overeat" is in quotes because it is relative—i.e., eating more than a diet allows does not necessarily mean you ate more than your body needed.

Diet Culture Harms

Diet culture is built on a faulty foundation. Our body size is largely determined by genetics, not by how many calories we consume or burn at the gym. Diets are far more likely to lead to weight *gain* than sustainable weight loss, and repeated attempts to shrink our body are not beneficial for health. There is no one right way to eat, and there are a host of factors beyond nutrition and exercise that need to be considered for health. Relying on a diet's rules instead of trusting our body's wisdom is not a worthwhile accomplishment. A thinner body is not an indicator of a healthier body and certainly not a sign of virtue or superiority. Perhaps most importantly, our value does not come from our body size, shape, or appearance.

Diet culture harms in a multitude of ways including through the myths it perpetuates. By challenging these falsehoods, we can begin to loosen diet culture's hold.

You Can't Ignore Genetics

One of the most detrimental assumptions in diet culture is that we can choose the body we want to have, and if we follow the right diet and exercise plan, we can achieve it. If we don't reach our body goals, it's our fault—we didn't try hard enough, we didn't follow the program properly, or we didn't want it bad enough. Although behaviors and environmental factors play a role in our body weight and shape, research suggests that body size may be up to 80% attributable to genetics.[9] Biology also determines how your body reacts when you alter your eating. A significant increase in food intake will lead to weight gain in some people, and in others, weight will remain stable despite eating more.[8] Similarly, caloric restriction results in weight loss for some individuals, but not for everyone. Following the exact same diet and exercise program as someone you admire won't make your body look like theirs. Our genes are the main factor that influences our weight and shape, yet diet culture continues to perpetuate the myth that it's all about our willpower.

Diets Don't Work

Most people go on a diet because they want to lose weight or believe a diet will help them feel better about their body or will make them healthier. Although many diet plans lead to some weight loss in the first few weeks to months, the evidence is conclusive that diets don't work in the long term, and this has been known for decades. Over 60 years ago, research by Dr. Albert Stunkard found that very few people were able to lose significant weight on a diet, and among those who did, the majority regained most or all of what they lost. At the two-year follow-up for this study, only 2% of participants were successful in maintaining their weight loss.[10] In 1992, a National Institutes of Health (NIH) panel of experts found that most dieters regain up to two-thirds of lost weight within one year and almost all lost weight is regained within five years. They concluded that diets don't work,[11] which has been confirmed by numerous additional studies.[12,13]

According to Dr. Traci Mann, who has been researching dieting for over 20 years, diets are destined to fail. Biological changes (i.e., not a lack of willpower) that happen in the body when we diet, such as altered appetite hormones and a slower metabolism, make it basically impossible to keep off lost weight.[14] Dr. Mann and her colleagues found that one-third to two-thirds of dieters regained more weight than they lost (and the authors think this is likely an underestimate). So, not only do diets fail to lead to lasting weight loss, but dieting is actually a strong predictor of future weight gain.[12]

Weight-loss diets also fail to improve health. A few diet programs have been associated with slightly improved health markers (e.g., blood pressure, fasting blood sugar, cholesterol) but these changes weren't correlated with weight loss.[15] In other words, these improvements probably happened because the participants increased healthy behaviors such as exercise and eating more fiber.[15]

Dieting Isn't Healthy

Despite what diet culture would like you to believe, repeated attempts to shrink, shape, and trim your body into a smaller form than you are biologically meant to be are not without consequence. If you have been on a diet before or have been around a dieter, you're probably familiar with the feelings of deprivation and increased food preoccupation and hunger that accompany dieting. These are the ways that your body, wired for survival, encourages you to eat when faced with food restriction. Restricting what or how much you eat gives food greater reward value, making it more likely that you'll feel out of control with food (especially "forbidden" foods) and "overeat" or engage in binge eating. Not surprisingly, binge eating is more common among dieters than non-dieters.[16]

The inevitable cycle of going on/off a diet (see Figure 1.1) leads to feelings of shame and guilt and negatively affects mood, body image, and self-esteem. Weight-cycling—repeated weight loss and subsequent regain that is the typical outcome of dieting—is also associated with health concerns such as dyslipidemia, insulin resistance,[17] high blood pressure,[17,18] increased inflammation,[19] and a higher risk for diabetes, heart attack, stroke,[20] and death.[21]

Food restriction can lead to energy and nutrient deficiencies which negatively impact physical and mental health (consequences of under-fueling in dancers are discussed in detail in Chapter 2). Of particular concern is the well-established link between dieting and eating disorders. A study that followed adolescents over the span of three years found that female participants who engaged in severe dieting (i.e., very frequent use of behaviors such as calorie counting, eating less at meals, and skipping meals)[22] were 18 times more likely to develop an eating disorder than non-dieters, and those who dieted moderately (i.e., used dieting behaviors less frequently) were five times more likely to develop an eating disorder than those who did not diet.[23] Table 1.2 lists additional negative consequences of dieting.

Redefining Health

Many people believe that diet, weight, and exercise are the main factors that determine one's health. However, diet and exercise together with personal behaviors like smoking and alcohol and drug use are only a small part of what affects health.[32]

Table 1.2 Consequences of Dieting

Physical Health	Mental Health
Higher cortisol[24]	Increased psychological stress[24,25]
Slower metabolism[26,27]	Impaired cognitive performance[28]
Delayed growth and development[29]	Depression[30]
Poorer bone health[31]	Anxiety[22]
Fatigue[27]	Lower self-esteem[25]

Table 1.3 Social Determinants of Health

Occupation	Pollution and water quality	Education and literacy
Income	Childhood experiences	Social support
Food security	Trauma	Access to technology
Housing	Racism and discrimination	Access to quality health care
Transportation	Segregation	Health insurance
Crime and violence	Stress	Culture

Adapted from Centers for Disease Control and Prevention,[34] County Health Rankings & Roadmaps,[32] and World Health Organization.[35]

The circumstances people are born into; the conditions they live, grow, and work in; and the larger systems that impact their quality of life are known as the social determinants of health (see Table 1.3).[33] These interconnected issues and circumstances influence health and well-being more than lifestyle choices.[33] Diet culture doesn't acknowledge the key role that social determinants or genetics play in our health, instead placing all the blame for our health issues on our eating and exercise habits. Diet culture causes additional harm by promoting a Eurocentric, privileged, one-diet-fits-all approach that fails to account for individual needs, cultural preferences, and access to resources.

Your Body Is Wise

The human body is constantly sending messages—telling you if you might be in danger, hurt, or sick; and when you need to eat, drink, rest, and go to the bathroom. Tuning in and honoring these cues is an important aspect of health. Yet, diet culture makes us question and judge the valuable signals our body is sending. Why am I hungry? I shouldn't be hungry. It's too early to eat lunch. Why am I so lazy? I need to make myself go to the gym.

When you're on a diet, you're expected to ignore your body's cues and trick yourself into consuming less than you need (e.g., "drink water before meals to help you feel full"). Diets rely on a set of rules and restrictions to determine when, what, and how much to eat, which impairs the ability to intuitively regulate your intake.[27] Dismissing your body's hunger (and other) cues breaks body trust. When you don't trust your body's messages and your body doesn't trust you to care for it, health can suffer.

Our Kids Are Not Alright

Diet culture begins to exert its harmful influence on children at a young age. An estimated 40–50% of 6–12-year-olds experience body dissatisfaction,[36] and participation in aesthetic sports (including dance) has been shown to increase weight concerns in girls as young as five years old.[37] An older study found that more than 60% of fourth graders "very often" or "sometimes" wished they were thinner and worried about being fat, and about

40% reported going on a diet "very often" or "sometimes." Among the same 9–11-year-old children, over 80% reported that a family member was "very often" or "sometimes" on a diet,[38] highlighting the influence of environment. Because of when this research was conducted, it doesn't capture the impact of social media use which has been repeatedly linked to body dissatisfaction, dieting, and disordered eating in pre-teens and adolescents (and young adults).[39–41] Of note, desire for weight loss and dieting behaviors are common in adolescents who are of "normal" weight and even present in those who are "underweight."[22,42,43]

Children aren't afforded the opportunity to develop their identity and sense of self-worth separate from the influence of diet culture. And, as discussed in the Dancing in Diet Culture section below, the dance environment is likely to exacerbate the effects of diet culture. Considering that many dancers begin training at a very young age and, at higher levels, are spending multiple hours a day in the dance environment, it's understandable that the impact on their body image and eating can be profound and enduring.

Diet culture harms through the value and privilege it ascribes to thinness/leanness. Diet culture standards have always served to exclude—drawing a line between the acceptable and worthy and the unacceptable and less valuable. With so much at stake, it's no wonder that, despite the health risks and well-documented failure rate of dieting, we are lured into trying diet after diet, longing for a body that matches the one deemed ideal. I've had clients tell me that they would rather be sick or feel miserable than exist in a larger body. This is the power of diet culture's influence.

The Weight of Stigma

The darker side of our society's idealization of and preference for thin bodies is the harm perpetuated toward individuals in larger bodies. Weight stigma—also known as weight bias—refers to negative weight-based attitudes and beliefs that manifest in stereotypes, prejudice, and discrimination against higher-weight individuals.[44] Weight stigma shows up just about everywhere—in schools, the workplace, healthcare settings, interpersonal relationships, the media,[45] and in the dance world. Because weight bias is pervasive in our society, it can unwittingly become ingrained in all of us (even those of us who are actively working to combat it).

Individuals report feeling stigmatized most often by family members, doctors, and classmates.[46] Weight stigma may be blatant—like weight-related jokes/teasing, body shaming, social exclusion, bullying, or harassment—or it might be more subtle, such as giving unsolicited weight-loss advice or making assumptions about a person's capabilities or behaviors based on their body size or shape.[47,48] For example, it is often presumed that a dancer whose body is larger than the "ideal" desired by their school or company is "overeating." They may be instructed to reduce their food intake or exercise more, without an evaluation of or regard for whether the dancer may already be undereating, over-exercising, or have an eating disorder.

Regardless of the form it takes, weight stigma harms. People in larger bodies frequently face discrimination in employment settings—they are less likely to be hired or promoted than thinner individuals with the same qualifications, and they are paid less for doing the same job as their thinner coworkers.[45] This bias has a direct impact on a person's livelihood. Weight bias is also prevalent in healthcare settings. A review by Puhl and Heuer found that healthcare professionals across various disciplines (e.g., doctors, nurses, dietitians, psychologists) frequently believe weight-based stereotypes, have negative attitudes toward individuals at higher weights, and blame their patient's weight on poor lifestyle choices and lack of motivation and willpower rather than considering genetic or environmental causes.[49] These biases exist even among providers who specialize in treating eating disorders and "obesity."[48]

Attempts to justify anti-fat bias are often based on the assumption that being in a larger body is a health risk. However, many of the health problems blamed on higher weight might instead be due to weight stigma. Facing stigma is a major stressor, and this increased stress may explain why higher weights are often associated with poorer health.[50] Allostatic load—the cumulative adverse effects that repeated stress has on multiple body systems—is a strong predictor of chronic disease.[51] One long-term study found that participants who experienced weight-based discrimination were more than twice as likely to have high allostatic load than individuals who did not report weight discrimination.[51] Another study found that weight-based discrimination explained a notable proportion of the association between "obesity" and markers of poorer health.[52]

Weight stigma is also associated with multiple mental health concerns including depression, anxiety, low self-esteem, body dissatisfaction, suicidal thoughts, and disordered eating.[45] Disrespectful treatment and shaming are not effective ways to promote behavior change or improve health. In fact, experiencing weight stigma is linked to increased caloric consumption, feeling more out of control with food,[53] eating to cope,[46] and avoiding exercise.[54]

The linking of weight and health is much more controversial and complicated than the medical community and diet culture would like you to believe. Medical professionals, researchers, and insurance companies typically use body mass index (BMI) to decide if an individual has a "healthy" weight. This weight-to-height ratio was originally developed in the early 19th century by Belgian astronomer and mathematician Adolphe Quetelet to assess weights across a population. He was trying to statistically define the "average man" and never intended for BMI (then known as the Quetelet index) to be used clinically or to be a measure of body composition or an indicator of health.[55]

Nevertheless, Ancel Keys, a researcher who was quite open about his anti-fat bias,[3] felt it was necessary to have an easy way to estimate body fatness, and he decided BMI could be used to do so even though he stated that it was "not fully satisfactory" as an indicator of "obesity."[56] The idea that the health of individuals across genders, races, ethnicities, and ages can be determined by a universally applied math formula never intended for this purpose seems absurd, especially considering that the research supporting the use of this formula was based on all-male, presumably mostly White subjects. Yet, thanks in large part to Keys, using BMI as a marker of health and a means of pathologizing bodies was widely adopted, and its use remains pervasive today.

In addition, the cut-offs for "overweight" and "obese" classifications based on BMI are subjective and arbitrary at best and motivated to serve the interests of the pharmaceutical companies at worst.[57] Conflicts of interest in "obesity" research and policy are important to consider. As J. Eric Oliver states in his book *Fat Politics*:

> It is difficult to find any major figure in the field of obesity research or past president of the North American Association for the Study of Obesity who does not have some type of financial tie to a pharmaceutical or weight-loss company.[57]

If researchers, health and life insurance companies, medical providers, and the diet industry benefit from the notion that being "overweight" is unhealthy and that it's your fault if your body doesn't fit their definition of "ideal," it's no wonder we are bombarded with these messages. You're much less likely to hear about the research showing that "overweight" individuals have a lower risk of death than those of "normal" weight, and those with "grade 1 obesity" (i.e., BMI of 30 to < 35) have the same mortality risk as people in the "normal" weight category.[58] Diet culture certainly isn't broadcasting the research showing that stigmatizing people for their weight harms their health.

Because weight bias remains socially acceptable, it goes mostly unchallenged and unchecked.[59] Weight stigma disproportionately harms those in larger bodies, but it impacts everyone. Dancers of any body size may turn society's harmful attitudes and stereotypes about weight inward. This internalized weight bias affects how a dancer feels and behaves, particularly if they perceive themselves as "overweight." For example, dancers often have significant fear and shame about weight gain (even when it is expected and necessary such as in puberty), which may lead them to diet or engage in disordered eating. Weight bias may also impact the medical care a dancer gets, like when concerns about missed periods are dismissed because a dancer's weight is "normal."

Himmelstein and colleagues designed an interesting experiment to test the effects of being exposed to weight stigma. Participants were told they couldn't participate in a shopping activity because their body size and shape weren't ideal for the style of clothing. The women who believed themselves to be "heavy" had sustained elevations of cortisol (a stress hormone), whereas those who considered themselves of "normal" weight returned to their baseline level of cortisol after the stigmatizing event (of note, 50% of the participants who thought they were "heavy" had a BMI in the "normal" range). As the authors state, "these findings underscore the importance of self-perception in the experience of stigma."[60] Other studies have also found that simply perceiving oneself as "overweight" or wanting to lose weight takes a toll on physical and mental health, regardless of actual body size.[53,61] It's not hard to see how dancers who believe their bodies are larger than "ideal" can experience the negative health consequences of weight stigma.

Dancing in Diet Culture

The dance world exists within a larger world entrenched in diet culture. Dancers and their teachers, parents, and healthcare providers are all influenced by its messages and belief systems: a thinner dancer is a better dancer; there is a "right" and "wrong" way for dancers to eat; controlling food intake and body size are virtues and expectations of the profession; and, with enough discipline and hard work, a dancer can achieve an "ideal" body. Diet culture in dance can be so ingrained and accepted that its presence and impact are rarely questioned or addressed. The effect on dancers is significant and multifold. Dancers are directly exposed to these messages, affecting their self-evaluation and their behaviors. And those who train, employ, and care for dancers, often former dancers themselves, have internalized these beliefs, which influences how they view and work with dancers.

The dance world doesn't just reinforce diet culture's messages, it magnifies and amplifies them.[§] Body "ideals" in dance are even narrower than those in society, particularly in certain genres (e.g., ballet, modern, contemporary, Broadway). Although these body "ideals" are often explained as part of the tradition of dance or a necessary requirement to perform the art as it is "meant to be" done, a look through photos of dance icons from past decades challenges this justification. Dancers today require higher levels of athleticism to perform increasingly demanding choreography, and there appears to be more acceptance of an athletic build, though not all athletic body types are considered appropriate—the body must still be lean. Overall, body "ideals" in dance, like in our society, have shifted toward an ultra-thin physique that is now favored in much of the dance world.

Diet culture tells us that thinner bodies are more deserving of status, privilege, and praise than larger bodies, and this message is ever-present in dance. There are countless examples of thinner dancers getting selected for jobs, promotions, and featured roles over dancers with bodies that don't meet the thin ideal. Participation in certain classes, rehearsals, and performances as well as employment contracts may be contingent upon a dancer losing weight or maintaining a specified weight. Explanations for the weight requirements might include: the dancer needs to fit an existing costume which would be too expensive to alter or that girls/women need to be ultra-thin so that the boys/men don't get hurt doing lifts. Finances are a genuine concern in the arts, and we want the health of all dancers to be considered. But what do these explanations say about the value given to dancers' health and the ways in which gender hierarchies influence the priority given to protecting it?

Thankfully, recent attention to the harms of weigh-ins and body-shaming has made these practices somewhat less ubiquitous in the dance world than before, but they are far from extinct. Explicitly telling dancers to lose weight is also not considered as acceptable as it once was, so more schools and companies have shifted their language. They may tell dancers that they need to "tone-up," "get fit," or "lengthen." This veiled language is confusing (e.g., if a dancer with excellent strength, endurance, and other aspects of fitness is told to "get fit"), and most dancers hear these euphemisms as "My body is not okay as it is, and weight loss is needed to make it better."

Sometimes the request for weight loss comes with an additional directive, "we want you to do it the healthy way." Although it might be well-meaning, it is difficult to hear this statement as actual concern for the dancer's health, especially considering how frequently weight loss is praised and rewarded without knowing what the dancer is doing to lose weight or what other circumstances might be contributing to a lower weight (e.g., depression or a traumatic event). Dancers are often not given resources or professional guidance on what "healthy weight loss" means, and perhaps more importantly, if it is even possible. The words may say "we care about your health," but the environment consistently reinforces the message that a dancer's body size is more important than their health.

Pressure to have the "ideal" dance body is compounded by the fact that "ideal" is not just about body size. Although there is variability in preferred body type based on genre, many dancers are expected to have beautifully arched feet, long arms and legs, a short torso, a long neck, correct shoulder-to-hip proportions, and a small head—plus be flexible and have good turn-out.** Binary gender norms commonplace in dance also dictate body ideals. For female dancers, a pre-pubescent body lacking the breasts and hips characteristic of adult development is often preferred. Male dancers are expected to have six-pack abs and be strong, but not bulky. The body is an essential part of the art of dance, but with so much focus on meeting these "ideals," dancers can feel that their bodies are the most important thing about them—more valuable than their other qualities as artists and humans.

The highly competitive environment in dance further raises the stakes. Very few dancers are accepted to elite training schools and even fewer dance professionally. Many dancers (especially girls/women) have heard some version of "there are hundreds of dancers with just as much talent waiting in the wings to take your place." Dancers know they are replaceable. Dispensable. In this setting, the pressure to meet the aesthetic preferences of their school or company is intense. Make it or break it.

Dancers spend hours every day scrutinizing their bodies in the mirror in a competitive atmosphere—measuring their qualities against the extensive list of requirements necessary to achieve the "ideal" dancer body and comparing themselves to others. Dancers feel their bodies under constant surveillance and scrutiny by those in power.[1] There may be little reprieve from these pressures, particularly for dancers training and living away from their family or for those who rarely spend time with non-dance friends or participating in non-dance activities.

Feeling pressure to be thin is a strong predictor of body dissatisfaction,[62] and, as we might expect, body dissatisfaction is common among dancers across different genres.[63-66] Internalizing the thin ideal also contributes to increased body dissatisfaction.[62] The more unattainable the ideal, the more a dancer's body image may suffer. Body pressures can vary based on gender and dance genre, which may explain why more positive body image has been reported among some female modern dancers,[67] female contemporary dancers,[68] and male dancers.[69]

Body dissatisfaction is a known risk factor for developing an eating disorder.[62] When dancers are unhappy with their bodies, and especially when they believe their weight affects their performance,[70] they are more likely to engage in weight-loss behaviors.[70-72] Additionally, many preferred body traits in dance are unchangeable, so dancers may focus on areas that are seemingly more in their control. "I don't have great feet or extension, but at least I'm thin." "I can't control my environment, but I can try to control my body."

The use of harmful weight control methods (most of which are disordered eating behaviors) such as self-induced vomiting; using laxatives, diet pills, and diuretics; smoking; excessive exercise; skipping meals; fasting; and following restrictive fad diets are frequently reported by dancers.[63-66,70,71,73] Because disordered eating behaviors are normalized in diet culture and in dance, these harmful habits are often not identified as problematic. Negative body image is also associated with depression and anxiety,[30,72] which independently affect dancers' health and are additional risk factors for eating disorders.

The diet-culture belief that if you aren't getting the results you want, you just need to work harder feeds into the dancer mindset. Dancers are often perfectionists with tremendous discipline. They excel at working hard and denying the pain and discomfort that accompany the relentless drive to achieve their goals. The qualities that make them good dancers also make them vulnerable to the dangers of dieting. Dancers are willing to do whatever it takes to live their dream, but they shouldn't be required to sacrifice their health. From the moment a young dancer steps into a studio to the final bow of their career, the dance world teaches dancers about how they derive their worth and what caring for their body means. The impact of these explicit and implicit lessons is enduring, and the negative effects of the thin ideal in dance persist long after a dancer has stopped dancing.[74]

Roots Matter: Diet Culture × Racism × Dance

Diet culture's history is firmly rooted in racism,[††] classism, and sexism.[3,5,75] Our society's preference for thinner bodies comes from made-up hierarchies that originated hundreds of years ago. For centuries, those in positions of power categorized other humans in a way that served them—using it as a means to rationalize the exploitation and oppression of groups they deemed inferior and less civilized.[75] During the 1800s, an updated human hierarchical system emerged in the U.S. spurred by a surge of "undesirable" immigrants arriving from southern and eastern Europe.[3] Based on racial and evolutionary theories that applied similar constructs as those used to justify slavery, this system ranked humans based on race,[‡‡] gender, and physical attributes.[3,5,75] Not coincidentally, those creating the classifications put their own "type" at the highest rank.[5,75] As Amy Erdman Farrell writes:

> White, northern European cultures were at the top of the hierar-chy, African and Native American at the bottom, Asian and south-ern European in the middle. … [W]ithin each of these groups females clearly existed a step down from whatever heights of civilization their male brethren could reach.[75]

These hierarchies classified physical traits to provide "proof" of lower value as a human. Darker skin color and fatness were among the attributes that marked a person as inferior.[75] Within this spectrum of White equals good and Black equals bad, thinness (and eating restraint) was linked to Whiteness and fatness (and gluttony and other undesirable qualities) to Blackness.[3,75] Regarding gender, women were thought to be more prone to fatness than men, which served as "evidence" that women deserved their lower status.[75] By the early 20th century, thinness (particularly for women) was increas-ingly associated with wealth and privilege.[76] A slender (White) body differed from the physical stereotypes assigned to African Americans and immigrants and provided an outward sign of a person who did not need to be part of the working class.[76] Understanding diet culture's roots matters because anti-fatness is inextricably connected to a societal construct engineered to uphold White supremacy, classism, and patriarchy. By subscribing to and reinforcing the notion that thinner is better, we (consciously or unconsciously, deliber-ately or inadvertently) perpetuate an oppressive belief system and the harm it causes.

The impact of these centuries-old, pseudo-scientific racial theories can still be found in dance today, particularly in "Western" concert dance forms like ballet and modern.[77] As Crystal U. Davis and Jesse Phillips-Fein write, "Dance terminology, technique, curriculum, and pedagogy reflect values ascribed through Whiteness to corporeality and extend to the perception of bodies themselves."[77] A dancer demonstrates the control they have over their body through the mastery of technique and by molding their body into the "ideal" dancer form, presumably through hard work, discipline, and eating restraint. Bodies that don't conform to the "ideal" are assumed to be less civilized, undisciplined, and less deserving (the very same notions used by racial theorists to designate Black, Indigenous, and other bodies of color as inferior), so their exclusion from dance can be justified.[77] The body is used to designate as Other.[78]

Dancers' bodies come in all shapes, sizes, and skin colors with as much variability within a so-called racial category as there is between different ethnicities.[78] Yet, historically, Black dancers have been considered less "suitable" to perform certain types of dance (e.g., ballet, modern) and certain roles based on physical stereotypes (e.g., prominent buttocks, flat feet, limited turnout, bulky musculature), whether present or not.[78] Although dancers such as Janet Collins, Arthur Mitchell, Raven Wilkinson, Judith Jamison (plus many more)[79] and internationally renowned companies like Dance Theatre of Harlem and Alvin Ailey American Dance Theater long ago dispelled the myth of unsuitability based on race and skin color, the residue of these stereotypes remains. Even today, the exclusion of dancers of color is supported by the supposed need to maintain an aesthetic of uniformity—i.e., darker skin and curly or "frizzy" hair would be too distracting.[77,78] Of course, dancers of color wouldn't "stand out" if there was more diversity in dance. If dance is to thrive, the art form needs to expand who and what we see onstage to reflect our society and to be meaningful and enjoyable to more diverse audiences.

Expectations of how a dancer's body should look are influenced by a dance culture steeped in racism and diet culture, which has shaped the value ascribed to dancers' bodies. The closer a dancer of color's body is to the thin ideal—i.e., the more they embody the White European aesthetic—the fewer barriers they are likely to experience in the dance world.[78,80] However, aesthetic preferences are not the same thing as requirements to perform the art form at its highest levels. As Brenda Dixon Gottschild writes in her book *The Black Dancing Body*, "no dancing body—black, brown, or white—is inherently unfit for any kind of dance … It's really more about what we like to see than what the dancing body can be taught to do." And we must consider where we draw the line between preference and prejudice.[78]

The way racial stereotypes seemingly fit into traditional gender roles in dance is also at play. As Nyama McCarthy-Brown writes in "Dancing in the Margins: Experiences of African American Ballerinas," stereotypes associated with Black females (e.g., the "strong black woman") are not easily assimilated into a culture in which the ballerina is expected to appear ethereal, demure, and fragile[81] (which is also ironic considering the strength and athleticism required to be a ballerina). By contrast, Black male stereotypes (e.g., the "super performer") work more easily within ballet's confines.[81] According to Theresa Ruth Howard, Black male bodies are viewed as more acceptable because the role of the male ballet dancer "has always been in service to his ballerina. Since the white eye is accustomed to seeing the black male body in that station, it fits the stereotype of the black subservient laborer (he hauls, lifts, supports, fawns)."[82] For this reason, as well as the high demand for male dancers compared to females, male dancers of color may encounter fewer obstacles in their training and career than female dancers of color,[81] though stereotypes still impact casting decisions (e.g., biases may interfere with Black male dancers being seen as suited for the role of a Prince).

The impact of "stereotype threat" is important to consider as well. Psychologists Claude Steele and Joshua Aronson coined this term to describe the social-psychological predicament that arises when there are widely known negative stereotypes about some aspect of one's identity (e.g., race, gender, etc.). In these situations, there is a threat of being judged and treated according to that stereotype as well as pressure to not confirm the stereotype.[83,84] Steele and his colleagues found that students' academic performance suffered when they were confronted with a negative stereotype about their group. For example, when the researchers gave Black and White college students a test with difficult questions from the verbal Graduate Record Examination (GRE), Black students scored lower than White students when they were told that the exam measured intellectual ability but scored the same as White students when told the exam was a problem-solving task unrelated to ability.[83,84] Stereotype threat has a greater effect on those who care about and identify with the domain in which they are being stereotyped.[84]

Stereotypes can be destructive—not only in academics, but also in dance. In addition to impairing performance, stereotype threat can lead to disidentifying with the area of interest and decrease motivation to succeed.[84] A dancer under constant pressure to disprove stereotypes against them and who faces constant messages that they don't belong or aren't "right" for ballet, may doubt the possibility of a future in dance. The dancer might lose the drive to prove that they do have a place in ballet and may stop identifying as a dancer. How many gifted artists are we losing because of stereotypes in the dance world?

Racism and discrimination in dance appear in covert and blatant ways. Pink shoes and tights and straight hair slicked into a bun as the default for women in ballet. Black ballet dancers automatically encouraged to audition for the Alvin Ailey school or company.[80,85] Dancers of color being told they don't have the "right" body for ballet.[86] Artistic directors' preference for Black dancers with lighter skin.[82] Dancers of color given the slave, maid, thief, or "exotic" roles, but not cast as the Prince or Princess.[87,88] Dancers of color being used in marketing materials but not featured in casting.[88,89] Ballet productions using blackface.[90] Black dancers asked to powder (i.e., whiten) their skin for performances.[91,92] Popular dance works with offensive racial caricatures (e.g., the Chinese variation in *The Nutcracker*).

In an environment in which dancers of color must overcome multiple stereotypes, biases, and barriers, the pressure to achieve the thin ideal intensifies. In 2021, I co-presented a panel discussion for the International Conference on Eating Disorders on the role the lack of diversity, equity, and inclusion (DEI) in ballet plays in eating disorder development.[93] Our exploration of this topic included lived experiences of dancers via video interviews and from American Ballet Theatre principal dancer, Misty Copeland, who was a member of our presenting panel. Samuel Akins, a Black male ballet dancer, shared this powerful message[§§] about the intersection of race and the thin ideal in dance:

> Doing auditions, as sad as this is to say, [I don't want] the director to think about anything else but my dancing. And especially being a Black dancer, having that extra variable, I don't want my body to be a part of that. So, if my body is something that I know I can change to their liking, and I can't change my skin color, that takes away one extra variable that could be against me when they are ticking things off. When I am trying to prepare for these auditions, how do I look in the most balletic form? If we're just being point blank—thin. If I'm as thin as they would like me to be, or as in shape as they would like me to be, then my technique hopefully will be the only thing that they're looking at.

Notably, Akins takes on the burden of others' discrimination when that responsibility should fall to the directors, choreographers, and leadership.

Racism and discrimination compromise dancer health. A study by Langdon and Petracca found that non-White female dancers had more negative body image than White female dancers.[67] As mentioned previously, body dissatisfaction and pressure to attain the thin ideal can lead to harmful dieting practices and are risk factors for developing an eating disorder. In addition, racial discrimination is associated with other negative mental and physical health outcomes such as depression, anxiety, lower self-esteem, higher blood pressure, and inflammation.[94] Experiencing discrimination is also associated with alcohol consumption, cigarette smoking, and drug use in adolescents and adults.[94]

In a 2020 interview with *Pointe* magazine, dancer Chloé Lopes Gomes spoke about the racial discrimination and harassment she reportedly faced while dancing with Staatsballett Berlin. She says:

> I was so anxious and unwell that I ended up with a metatarsal fracture. I should have been back after two months, but six months later, I was still in pain, and the doctors didn't know why—until a neurologist told me it was linked to stress and prescribed antidepressants. Suddenly, the pain went away completely.[95]

Wouldn't it be great if the environment had changed?

Aesha Ash, former New York City Ballet (NYCB) dancer and current Associate Chair of Faculty at the School of American Ballet (SAB), in 2020 became the first Black woman appointed to SAB's permanent faculty.[96] As a dancer with NYCB, Ash says, "I was trying to battle stereotypes and biases on that stage every single night."[96] During most of her time in the company, she was the only Black female dancer, an isolating experience in which she felt excluded and Othered.[80] Racist comments—thinly veiled and overt—(e.g., that her body was "distracting") took their toll.[96] As Ash told the *New*

York Times, "That's talking to who you are. That chips away at your identity and your self-worth as a young adolescent coming into yourself, away from your home and away from your culture." Ash eventually decided to leave the company.[96]

In recent years the dance world has made strides in improving DEI. An increasing number of schools and companies now have initiatives dedicated to this effort, including expanding recruitment to underserved communities. The dance landscape is starting to shift. The number of dancers of color on some company rosters is gradually increasing. Black dance faculty, like Ash, are being hired at predominantly White institutions, and we are slowly beginning to see more diversity in leadership positions.[97] While it's important to acknowledge this progress, we cannot get comfortable as the dance world still has a long way to go. It's also vital to amplify and support the invaluable and continuing contributions that dance organizations of color (e.g., Dance Theatre of Harlem, Alvin Ailey American Dance Theater, Ballet Hispánico, Complexions Contemporary Ballet) make to the art form.

Challenging biases about dancers of color and confronting the impacts of racism and discrimination are essential to making the dance world a healthier and safer place. Dancers need equitable and inclusive access to training and safe spaces where they can thrive as artists and humans. According to C. S'thembile West:

> [D]ance educators have myriad opportunities to deconstruct, debunk, resist, dismantle, and transform the … mistruths about black and brown bodies. In an effort not to "dismiss" children of color in dance settings, dance pedagogues must address the beliefs, values, and attitudes that permeate social structures and impact the lives of students who enter dance classrooms and studios.[98]

Change begins with dance teachers and leadership acknowledging, evaluating, and challenging unconscious and conscious biases which can have a profound impact on a dancer's training and future—from the feedback they are given to the dance genres and careers they are encouraged to pursue (or not pursue).[77]

From ballet to modern to jazz and beyond, the dance environment should be a place that embraces different cultural identities and nurtures a sense of belonging that goes beyond just having one or two dancers of color in a school, company, or production. Addressing the socioeconomic factors that serve as additional barriers to diversity in dance is necessary. Dance training is expensive. One conservative calculation estimates that 15 years of ballet training will cost over $100,000.[99] Even dancers who are given tuition scholarships may face other challenges including the costs of dance shoes and attire; difficulty getting transportation to classes, rehearsals, performances, or competitions; and managing expectations of family involvement—not to mention all the additional costs if a dancer is training away from home.

Socioeconomic differences can make dancers feel Othered and that they don't have a place in dance.

Representation is key. Dancers of all colors, ethnicities, and backgrounds deserve to have teachers, role models, mentors, and leaders with similar identities to support and guide them. As Lydia Abarca-Mitchell, founding company member of Dance Theatre of Harlem, said when interviewed by Nyama McCarthy-Brown, "you need to be in an environment that you're gonna be nourished, loved, encouraged, choreographed upon and appreciated for all that you bring."[81] Dancers and the dance world need this—the future of the art form depends on it.

A Pause for Self-Compassion

Given the insidious nature of diet culture, the power of its influence, and the fact that most of us have been exposed to its messages for our entire lives, it makes sense that we might have unwittingly come to buy what diet culture has been selling. It's important to have compassion for ourselves as we confront the harms of diet culture and the part we may have inadvertently played in perpetuating them.

Diet culture and the narrow body ideals that exist in much of the dance world damage dancers by reducing their worth to their body and making them feel not good enough. Continually striving for improvement is an essential part of being a dancer, but when self-esteem, self-worth, and confidence suffer, so does expression, artistry, and growth as a dancer. How many talented dancers are we keeping from sharing their gifts because they fall just outside of the current dancer body "ideal"? What might happen if we each compassionately and non-judgmentally explored our own biases about dancers' bodies?

Because diet culture is a belief system, you can make the decision to stop believing in it. You can be a part of dismantling the influence and harms of diet culture—in dance and beyond. Acts II and III will provide guidance on ways to do so.

Main Pointes

- Diets don't work—they harm physical and mental health and are far more likely to lead to weight gain than sustainable weight loss.
- Thinner does not mean healthier.
- Dancers who diet are much more likely to develop an eating disorder.
- BMI is not a good indicator of health and should not be used to determine if a dancer is at a "healthy" weight.
- Weight stigma impacts everyone, but disproportionately harms people in larger bodies.
- Perceiving yourself as "overweight" and/or wanting to lose weight can negatively impact physical and mental health, regardless of actual body size.

- Body dissatisfaction is common among dancers and is a risk factor for dieting and eating disorder development.
- Preferences for and beliefs about how a dancer's body "should" look are heavily influenced by a dance culture steeped in diet culture and racism.
- Racism and discrimination compromise dancer health.
- Challenging stereotypes and biases about dancers of color and confronting the impacts of racism and discrimination are essential to making the dance world a healthier and safer place.

Notes

Close your eyes and imagine a ballet dancer. A modern dancer. A commercial dancer, Broadway dancer, hip-hop dancer. What do these dancers look like (body type, gender, skin color, hair, ethnicity)? Are there any stereotypes you might benefit from challenging?

What biases have you noticed in the dance world (in yourself and others)? How do you think these biases impact dancers and the art form?

Endnotes

* Pseudonym used in study.
† The books *Anti-Diet* by Christy Harrison and *Calories and Corsets* by Louise Foxcroft provide detailed histories of diet culture if you are interested in learning more.
‡ This weight-loss drug was banned five years after it hit the market because it was found to cause heart valve damage.[5]
§ Thankfully, several dance institutions are beginning to take steps toward recognizing and addressing some of this harmful traditional messaging.
** aka external rotation
†† Sabrina Strings' book, *Fearing the Black Body: The Racial Origins of Fat Phobia*, is an excellent resource on this topic.
‡‡ Race is a social construct.
§§ Edited lightly for readability.

References

1. Dryburgh A, Fortin S. Weighing in on surveillance: Perception of the impact of surveillance on female ballet dancers' health. *Res Dance Educ*. 2010;11(2):95–108. doi:10.1080/14647893.2010.482979
2. Tountas Y. The historical origins of the basic concepts of health promotion and education: The role of ancient Greek philosophy and medicine. *Health Promot Int*. 2009;24(2):185–192. doi:10.1093/heapro/dap006
3. Strings S. *Fearing the Black Body: The Racial Origins of Fat Phobia*. First ed. NYU Press; 2019:304.
4. Czerniawski AM. A 200-year weight debate. *Contexts*. 2017;16(3):68–69. doi:10.1177/1536504217732057

5. Harrison C. *Anti-Diet: Reclaim Your Time, Money, Well-Being, and Happiness Through Intuitive Eating.* First ed. Little, Brown Spark; 2019:336.
6. Naigaga DA, Jahanlu D, Claudius HM, Gjerlaug AK, Barikmo I, Henjum S. Body size perceptions and preferences favor overweight in adult Saharawi refugees. *Nutr J.* 2018;17(1):17. doi:10.1186/s12937-018-0330-5
7. Swami V, Frederick DA, Aavik T, et al. The attractive female body weight and female body dissatisfaction in 26 countries across 10 world regions: Results of the international body project I. *Pers Soc Psychol Bull.* 2010;36(3):309–325. doi:10.1177/0146167209359702
8. Foxcroft L. *Calories and Corsets: A History of Dieting over Two Thousand Years.* Main. Profile Books; 2012:241.
9. Nan C, Guo B, Warner C, et al. Heritability of body mass index in pre-adolescence, young adulthood and late adulthood. *Eur J Epidemiol.* 2012;27(4):247–253. doi:10.1007/s10654-012-9678-6
10. Stunkard A. The results of treatment for obesity. *AMA Arch Intern Med.* 1959;103(1):79. doi:10.1001/archinte.1959.00270010085011
11. Methods for voluntary weight loss and control. NIH Technology Assessment Conference Panel. *Ann Intern Med.* 1992;116(11):942–949. doi:10.7326/0003-4819-116-11-942
12. Mann T, Tomiyama AJ, Westling E, Lew A-M, Samuels B, Chatman J. Medicare's search for effective obesity treatments: Diets are not the answer. *Am Psychol.* 2007;62(3):220–233. doi:10.1037/0003-066X.62.3.220
13. Loveman E, Frampton GK, Shepherd J, et al. The clinical effectiveness and cost-effectiveness of long-term weight management schemes for adults: A systematic review. *Health Technol Assess.* 2011;15(2):1–182. doi:10.3310/hta15020
14. Ferdman RA. Why diets don't actually work, according to a researcher who has studied them for decades. *The Washington Post.* May 4, 2015. Accessed August 3, 2022. https://www.washingtonpost.com/news/wonk/wp/2015/05/04/why -diets-dont-actually-work-according-to-a-researcher-who-has-studied-them-for -decades/
15. Tomiyama AJ, Ahlstrom B, Mann T. Long-term effects of dieting: Is weight loss related to health? *Soc Personal Psychol Compass.* 2013;7(12):861–877. doi:10.1111/spc3.12076
16. Field AE, Austin SB, Taylor CB, et al. Relation between dieting and weight change among preadolescents and adolescents. *Pediatrics.* 2003;112(4):900–906. doi:10.1542/peds.112.4.900
17. Montani JP, Viecelli AK, Prévot A, Dulloo AG. Weight cycling during growth and beyond as a risk factor for later cardiovascular diseases: The "repeated overshoot" theory. *Int J Obes (Lond).* 2006;30(Suppl 4):S58–66. doi:10.1038/sj.ijo.0803520
18. Guagnano MT, Ballone E, Pace-Palitti V, et al. Risk factors for hypertension in obese women. The role of weight cycling. *Eur J Clin Nutr.* 2000;54(4):356–360. doi:10.1038/sj.ejcn.1600963
19. Strohacker K, McFarlin BK. Influence of obesity, physical inactivity, and weight cycling on chronic inflammation. *Front Biosci (Elite Ed).* 2010;2:98–104. doi:10.2741/e70
20. French SA, Folsom AR, Jeffery RW, Zheng W, Mink PJ, Baxter JE. Weight variability and incident disease in older women: The Iowa Women's Health Study. *Int J Obes Relat Metab Disord.* 1997;21(3):217–223. doi:10.1038/sj.ijo.0800390
21. Lissner L, Odell PM, D'Agostino RB, et al. Variability of body weight and health outcomes in the Framingham population. *N Engl J Med.* 1991;324(26):1839–1844. doi:10.1056/NEJM199106273242602

22. Patton GC, Carlin JB, Shao Q, et al. Adolescent dieting: Healthy weight control or borderline eating disorder? *J Child Psychol & Psychiat.* 1997;38(3):299–306. doi:10.1111/j.1469-7610.1997.tb01514.x

23. Patton GC, Selzer R, Coffey C, Carlin JB, Wolfe R. Onset of adolescent eating disorders: Population based cohort study over 3 years. *BMJ.* 1999;318(7186):765–768. doi:10.1136/bmj.318.7186.765

24. Tomiyama AJ, Mann T, Vinas D, Hunger JM, Dejager J, Taylor SE. Low calorie dieting increases cortisol. *Psychosom Med.* 2010;72(4):357–364. doi:10.1097/PSY.0b013e3181d9523c

25. Polivy J, Heatherton T. Spiral model of dieting and disordered eating. In: Wade T, ed. *Encyclopedia of Feeding and Eating Disorders.* Springer Singapore; 2017:791–793. doi:10.1007/978-981-287-104-6_94

26. Kajioka T, Tsuzuku S, Shimokata H, Sato Y. Effects of intentional weight cycling on non-obese young women. *Metab Clin Exp.* 2002;51(2):149–154. doi:10.1053/meta.2002.29976

27. Herman CP, Polivy J. The self-regulation of eating: Theoretical and practical problems. In: *Handbook of Self-Regulation: Research, Theory, and Applications.* The Guilford Press; 2004:492–508.

28. Jones N, Rogers PJ. Preoccupation, food, and failure: An investigation of cognitive performance deficits in dieters. *Int J Eat Disord.* 2003;33(2):185–192. doi:10.1002/eat.10124

29. Pugliese MT, Lifshitz F, Grad G, Fort P, Marks-Katz M. Fear of obesity. A cause of short stature and delayed puberty. *N Engl J Med.* 1983;309(9):513–518. doi:10.1056/NEJM198309013090901

30. Stice E, Bearman SK. Body-image and eating disturbances prospectively predict increases in depressive symptoms in adolescent girls: A growth curve analysis. *Dev Psychol.* 2001;37(5):597–607. doi:10.1037//0012-1649.37.5.597

31. Van Loan MD, Keim NL. Influence of cognitive eating restraint on total-body measurements of bone mineral density and bone mineral content in premenopausal women aged 18–45 y: A cross-sectional study. *Am J Clin Nutr.* 2000;72(3):837–843. doi:10.1093/ajcn/72.3.837

32. County Health Rankings & Roadmaps. County health rankings model. Accessed August 10, 2022. https://www.countyhealthrankings.org/explore-health-rankings/measures-data-sources/county-health-rankings-model

33. World Health Organization. Social determinants of health. Accessed November 11, 2022. https://www.who.int/health-topics/social-determinants-of-health#tab=tab_1

34. Centers for Disease Control and Prevention. NCHHSTP social determinants of health. Accessed August 12, 2022. https://www.cdc.gov/nchhstp/socialdeterminants/faq.html

35. Wilkinson R, Marmot M. *Social Determinants of Health [OP]: The Solid Facts (Public Health).* 2nd ed. World Health Organization; 2003:31.

36. Cash TF, Smolak L. Body image development in childhood. In: *Body Image: A Handbook of Science, Practice, and Prevention.* 2nd ed. Guilford Press; 2011.

37. Davison KK, Earnest MB, Birch LL. Participation in aesthetic sports and girls' weight concerns at ages 5 and 7 years. *Int J Eat Disord.* 2002;31(3):312–317. doi:10.1002/eat.10043

38. Gustafson-Larson AM, Terry RD. Weight-related behaviors and concerns of fourth-grade children. *J Am Diet Assoc.* 1992;92(7):818–822. doi:10.1016/S0002-8223(21)00736-7

39. Wilksch SM, O'Shea A, Ho P, Byrne S, Wade TD. The relationship between social media use and disordered eating in young adolescents. *Int J Eat Disord.* 2020;53(1):96–106. doi:10.1002/eat.23198

40. Tiggemann M, Slater A. NetTweens. The internet and body image concerns in preteenage girls. *J Early Adolesc.* 2014;34(5):606–620. doi:10.1177/0272431613501083
41. Holland G, Tiggemann M. A systematic review of the impact of the use of social networking sites on body image and disordered eating outcomes. *Body Image.* 2016;17:100–110. doi:10.1016/j.bodyim.2016.02.008
42. Neumark-Sztainer D, Story M, Hannan PJ, Perry CL, Irving LM. Weight-related concerns and behaviors among overweight and nonoverweight adolescents. *Arch Pediatr Adolesc Med.* 2002;156(2):171. doi:10.1001/archpedi.156.2.171
43. Hijji TM, Saleheen H, AlBuhairan FS. Underweight, body image, and weight loss measures among adolescents in Saudi Arabia: Is it a fad or is there more going on? *Int J Pediatr Adolesc Med.* 2021;8(1):18–24. doi:10.1016/j.ijpam.2020.01.002
44. Puhl RM, Moss-Racusin CA, Schwartz MB, Brownell KD. Weight stigmatization and bias reduction: Perspectives of overweight and obese adults. *Health Educ Res.* 2008;23(2):347–358. doi:10.1093/her/cym052
45. Puhl RM, King KM. Weight discrimination and bullying. *Best Pract Res Clin Endocrinol Metab.* 2013;27(2):117–127. doi:10.1016/j.beem.2012.12.002
46. Puhl RM, Brownell KD. Confronting and coping with weight stigma: An investigation of overweight and obese adults. *Obesity (Silver Spring).* 2006;14(10):1802–1815. doi:10.1038/oby.2006.208
47. Neumark-Sztainer D, Story M, Faibisch L. Perceived stigmatization among overweight African-American and Caucasian adolescent girls. *J Adolesc Health.* 1998;23(5):264–270. doi:10.1016/s1054-139x(98)00044-5
48. Tylka TL, Annunziato RA, Burgard D, et al. The weight-inclusive versus weight-normative approach to health: Evaluating the evidence for prioritizing well-being over weight loss. *J Obes.* 2014;2014:983495. doi:10.1155/2014/983495
49. Puhl RM, Heuer CA. The stigma of obesity: A review and update. *Obesity (Silver Spring).* 2009;17(5):941–964. doi:10.1038/oby.2008.636
50. Muennig P. The body politic: The relationship between stigma and obesity-associated disease. *BMC Public Health.* 2008;8:128. doi:10.1186/1471-2458-8-128
51. Vadiveloo M, Mattei J. Perceived weight discrimination and 10-year risk of Allostatic load among US adults. *Ann Behav Med.* 2017;51(1):94–104. doi:10.1007/s12160-016-9831-7
52. Daly M, Sutin AR, Robinson E. Perceived weight discrimination mediates the prospective association between obesity and physiological dysregulation: Evidence from a population-based cohort. *Psychol Sci.* 2019;30(7):1030–1039. doi:10.1177/0956797619849440
53. Major B, Hunger JM, Bunyan DP, Miller CT. The ironic effects of weight stigma. *J Exp Soc Psychol.* 2014;51:74–80. doi:10.1016/j.jesp.2013.11.009
54. Vartanian LR, Shaprow JG. Effects of weight stigma on exercise motivation and behavior: A preliminary investigation among college-aged females. *J Health Psychol.* 2008;13(1):131–138. doi:10.1177/1359105307084318
55. Eknoyan G. Adolphe Quetelet (1796-1874)-the average man and indices of obesity. *Nephrol Dial Transplant.* 2008;23(1):47–51. doi:10.1093/ndt/gfm517
56. Keys A, Fidanza F, Karvonen MJ, Kimura N, Taylor HL. Indices of relative weight and obesity. *Int J Epidemiol.* 2014;43(3):655–665. doi:10.1093/ije/dyu058
57. Oliver JE. *Fat Politics: The Real Story behind America's Obesity Epidemic.* Illustrated. Oxford University Press; 2006:242.

58. Flegal KM, Kit BK, Orpana H, Graubard BI. Association of all-cause mortality with overweight and obesity using standard body mass index categories: A systematic review and meta-analysis. *JAMA*. 2013;309(1):71–82. doi:10.1001/jama.2012.113905

59. Puhl R. Weight discrimination: A socially acceptable injustice. Obesity Action Coalition. June 2008. Accessed August 17, 2022. https://www.obesityaction.org/resources/weight-discrimination-a-socially-acceptable-injustice/

60. Himmelstein MS, Incollingo Belsky AC, Tomiyama AJ. The weight of stigma: Cortisol reactivity to manipulated weight stigma. *Obesity (Silver Spring)*. 2015;23(2):368–374. doi:10.1002/oby.20959

61. Muennig P, Jia H, Lee R, Lubetkin E. I think therefore I am: Perceived ideal weight as a determinant of health. *Am J Public Health*. 2008;98(3):501–506. doi:10.2105/AJPH.2007.114769

62. Stice E, Whitenton K. Risk factors for body dissatisfaction in adolescent girls: A longitudinal investigation. *Dev Psychol*. 2002;38(5):669–678. doi:10.1037//0012-1649.38.5.669

63. Robbeson JG, Kruger HS, Wright HH. Disordered eating behavior, body image, and energy status of female student dancers. *Int J Sport Nutr Exerc Metab*. 2015;25(4):344–352. doi:10.1123/ijsnem.2013-0161

64. Anshel MH. Sources of disordered eating patterns between ballet dancers and non-dancers. *J Sport Behav*. 2004;27(2):115–133.

65. Santo André HC, Pinto AJ, Mazzolani BC, et al. "Can a Ballerina eat ice cream?": A mixed-method study on eating attitudes and body image in female ballet dancers. *Front Nutr*. 2021;8:665654. doi:10.3389/fnut.2021.665654

66. Heiland TL, Murray DS, Edley PP. Body image of dancers in Los Angeles: The cult of slenderness and media influence among dance students. *Res Dance Educ*. 2008;9(3):257–275. doi:10.1080/14647890802386932

67. Langdon SW, Petracca G. Tiny dancer: Body image and dancer identity in female modern dancers. *Body Image*. 2010;7(4):360–363. doi:10.1016/j.bodyim.2010.06.005

68. Swami V, Harris AS. Dancing toward positive body image? Examining body-related constructs with ballet and contemporary dancers at different levels. *Am J Dance Ther*. 2012;34(1):39–52. doi:10.1007/s10465-012-9129-7

69. Danis A, Jamaludin AN, Majid HA MohdA, Isa KAM. Body image perceptions among dancers in urban environmental settings. *Procedia Soc Behav Sci*. 2016;222:855–862. doi:10.1016/j.sbspro.2016.05.196

70. Gearhart MG, Sugimoto D, Meehan WP, Stracciolini A. Body satisfaction, performance perception, and weight loss behavior in young female dancers. *Med Probl Perform Art*. 2018;33(4):225–230. doi:10.21091/mppa.2018.4033

71. Hidayah GN, Bariah AHS. Eating attitude, body image, body composition and dieting behaviour among dancers. *Asian J Clin Nutr*. 2011;3(3):92–102. doi:10.3923/ajcn.2011.92.102

72. Arcelus J, García-Dantas A, Sánchez-Martín M, Río-Sanchez C. Influence of perfectionism on variables associated to eating disorders in dancers. *Rev Psicol Deporte*. 2015;24:297–303.

73. Thomas JJ, Keel PK, Heatherton TF. Disordered eating attitudes and behaviors in ballet students: Examination of environmental and individual risk factors. *Int J Eat Disord*. 2005;38(3):263–268. doi:10.1002/eat.20185

74. Ackard DM, Henderson JB, Wonderlich AL. The associations between childhood dance participation and adult disordered eating and related psychopathology. *J Psychosom Res*. 2004;57(5):485–490. doi:10.1016/j.jpsychores.2004.03.004

75. Farrell AE. Fat and the un-civilized body. In: *Fat Shame: Stigma and the Fat Body in American Culture.* NYU Press; 2011:59–81.
76. Jou C. The progressive era body project: Calorie-counting and "disciplining the stomach" in 1920s America. *J Gilded Age Prog Era.* 2019;18(4):422–440. doi:10.1017/S1537781418000348
77. Davis CU, Phillips-Fein J. Tendus and tenancy: Black dancers and the white landscape of dance education. In: Kraehe AM, Gaztambide-Fernández R, Carpenter II BS, eds. *The Palgrave Handbook of Race and the Arts in Education.* Springer International Publishing; 2018:571–584. doi:10.1007/978-3-319-65256-6_33
78. Gottschild BD. *The Black Dancing Body.* Palgrave Macmillan US; 2003. doi:10.1007/978-1-137-03900-2
79. MoBBallet. The constellation project: Mapping the dark stars of ballet. Accessed November 19, 2022. https://mobballet.org/TheConstellationProject/
80. Angyal C. *Turning Pointe: How a New Generation of Dancers Is Saving Ballet from Itself.* Bold Type Books; 2021:304.
81. McCarthy-Brown N. Dancing in the margins: Experiences of African American ballerinas. *J Afr Am St.* 2011;15(3):385–408. doi:10.1007/s12111-010-9143-0
82. Howard TR. Op-Ed: Is ballet "brown bagging" it? *Dance Magazine.* April 2, 2017. Accessed July 23, 2022. https://www.dancemagazine.com/is-ballet-brown-bagging-it/
83. Steele CM, Aronson J. Stereotype threat and the intellectual test performance of African Americans. *J Pers Soc Psychol.* 1995;69(5):797–811. doi:10.1037/0022-3514.69.5.797
84. Steele CM. A threat in the air. How stereotypes shape intellectual identity and performance. *Am Psychol.* 1997;52(6):613–629. doi:10.1037/0003-066X.52.6.613
85. Fentroy CM. My experience as a Black Ballerina in a world of implicit bias. *Pointe.* June 4, 2020. Accessed July 23, 2022. https://pointemagazine.com/chyrstyn-fentroy/
86. Brodsky S. Misty Copeland says coded language is used to keep black and brown dancers out of ballet. *Popsugar.* October 20, 2020. Accessed July 23, 2022. https://www.popsugar.com/fitness/misty-copeland-interview-on-body-image-racism-in-ballet-47865540
87. Porter II JM. Dancing towards the dream of Asian representation. *The Body.* May 28, 2021. Accessed July 23, 2022. https://www.thebody.com/article/dancing-towards-the-dream-of-asian-representation
88. Copeland C. Ballet companies confront increasingly urgent calls for racial justice. *Prism.* September 17, 2020. Accessed July 23, 2022. https://prismreports.org/2020/09/17/ballet-companies-confront-increasingly-urgent-calls-for-racial-justice/
89. Seibert B. Black in ballet: Coming together after trying to 'blend into the corps.' *The New York Times.* August 17, 2021. Accessed July 24, 2022. https://www.nytimes.com/2021/08/17/arts/dance/misty-copeland-little-island.html.
90. Anonymous. Russia's Bolshoi rejects Misty Copeland's "blackface" criticism. *BBC News.* December 16, 2019. Accessed July 23, 2022. https://www.bbc.com/news/world-europe-50807742
91. Howard TR. What the Staatsballett Berlin case tells us about the power of artistic staff. *Dance Magazine.* December 15, 2020. Accessed July 23, 2022. https://www.dancemagazine.com/chloe-lopes-gomes-racism/?rebelltitem=4#rebelltitem4
92. Alford NS. Misty Copeland was once told to lighten her skin for a ballet role. Why she said 'no.' February 26, 2019. Accessed November 20, 2022. https://

thegrio.com/2019/02/26/misty-copeland-was-once-told-to-lighten-her-skin-for
-a-ballet-role-why-she-said-no/

93. Gorrell S, Hower H, Saigal M, Somehara F, Copeland M. The Role of Lack of
Diversity, Equity, and Inclusion in Ballet: Learning from the past and present
to shape the future of eating disorder prevention and treatment in dancers.
Presented at the: International Conference on Eating Disorders (ICED); June
12, 2021.

94. Williams DR, Lawrence JA, Davis BA, Vu C. Understanding how
discrimination can affect health. *Health Serv Res*. 2019;54(Suppl 2):1374–
1388. doi:10.1111/1475-6773.13222

95. Cappelle L. Chloé Lopes Gomes speaks out about racial harassment at
Staatsballett Berlin. *Pointe*. November 30, 2020. Accessed July 29, 2022.
https://pointemagazine.com/chloe-lopes-gomes-ballet/

96. Kourlas G. Aesha Ash takes her place at the head of the class. *The New York
Times*. August 13, 2020. Accessed July 29, 2022. https://www.nytimes.com
/2020/08/13/arts/dance/aesha-ash-american-ballet-faculty.html

97. Kaufman SL. Black women are finally shattering the glass ceiling in dance.
August 18, 2021. Accessed November 20, 2022. https://www.phillytrib.com/
entertainment/black-women-are-finally-shattering-the-glass-ceiling-in-dance/
article_88ed2dab-73fd-59d9-a06d-e7791b325b8c.html

98. West CS. Black bodies in dance education: Charting a new pedagogical
paradigm to eliminate gendered and hypersexualized assumptions. *J Dance
Educ*. 2005;5(2):64–69. doi:10.1080/15290824.2005.10387287

99. Abrams A. Raising a Ballerina will cost you $100,000. *FiveThirtyEight*. August
20, 2015. Accessed July 29, 2022. https://fivethirtyeight.com/features/high-price
-of-ballet-diversity-misty-copeland/

2   Dancing on Empty

One cannot think well, love well, sleep well, if one has not dined well.
~Virginia Woolf [i]

Dancing While Depleted

Susan tries to stay a few hundred calories below the goal set by her tracking app. She mostly eats lean protein and vegetables at her meals and never adds oil or other fats.

After his recent move to the U.S., Matt stopped having milk, cheese, and yogurt because he doesn't like the taste of American dairy products. He occasionally puts almond milk in his cereal.

Aliyah follows the keto diet and does intermittent fasting. She wants to be healthy, so she takes supplements daily which include high-dose vitamin C; a hair, skin, and nails vitamin; a mega-women's multivitamin; vitamin B12; and an "energy-boosting" herb mix.

Neil isn't hungry in the morning, so he just has a coffee before class. He brings a turkey sandwich for lunch but doesn't always have time to finish it before afternoon rehearsal. He doesn't want to lose any weight—he's actually hoping to gain some muscle—so he makes sure to have a large balanced dinner and a substantial snack before bed.

Sophia wants to lose weight, but she keeps messing up on her new diet. She sticks to it during the dance day, eating only "good" foods at meals and no snacks. Once she gets home, she feels so hungry that she can't stop eating, sometimes even eating her roommate's cookies. She feels out of control, uncomfortably full, and horribly guilty after.

Susan, Matt, Aliyah, Neil, and Sophia illustrate some of the ways in which dancers' fueling practices may be less than optimal. Dancers like Susan who

---

i Reprinted with permission from Woolf, V. *A Room of One's Own* (Bradshaw D, Clarke SN, eds.). John Wiley & Sons, Ltd.; 2015:192.

DOI: 10.4324/9781003366171-3

aren't eating enough calories (aka energy) usually also have insufficient intakes of essential nutrients. Nutrient deficiencies also occur in dancers whose diets are adequate in energy but lack in variety or are poorly balanced. For example, Matt's diet is low in calcium, though he may be eating enough calories. Aliyah consumes excessive amounts of vitamins and minerals, but her diet is deficient in carbohydrates, and she has long gaps without sufficient fuel. Although for different reasons, Neil and Sophia are both dancing in an under-fueled state despite their higher intakes at night. To help dancers stay physically and mentally healthy and dance at their best, we need to identify and address any situations that lead to suboptimal fueling in dancers.

In this chapter, I use the terms "under-fueling," "under-eating," and "suboptimal or inadequate fueling" interchangeably when referring to any of the ways in which dancers may be consuming less energy and/or fewer nutrients than they need for optimal health and performance. Table 2.1 provides definitions for additional terms that will be used in this chapter.

Table 2.1 Chapter 2 Definitions

Amenorrhea	Absence of menstrual periods[1]
Bone mass	The amount of bone tissue in the body[2]
Bone mineral density (BMD)	The amount of minerals (mostly calcium and phosphorus) in bone in a given area.[2] An indicator of bone strength and quality.[3] Also known as bone density.
Energy availability	The amount of energy that's left over to fuel the body's needs after dietary energy (calories) has been used for exercise[4]
Energy deficiency	When energy intake is less than the amount needed for normal body functioning, health, growth/development, daily activities, and exercise.[5] Also known as low energy availability.
Functional hypothalamic amenorrhea	Absence of periods due to a hormonal imbalance caused by under-fueling, over-exercising, and/or stress[6]
Low energy availability (LEA)	When there isn't enough energy left over to fuel the body's needs after dietary energy has been used for exercise.[4] Some studies use a specific threshold (of calories per kilogram of fat-free mass per day) to define LEA, below which normal body functions are likely to be impaired. This threshold will not be covered in this book because the research is inconclusive and there is substantial variability based on individual factors.[5]
Menarche	First menstrual period
Osteoporosis	A disease that occurs when bone mass and density are diminished, changing the structure and quality of bone which results in weakened bones and increased fracture risk[7]
Peak bone mass	The maximum amount of bone a person can attain[8]

Prevalence of Under-Fueling

Decades of research have consistently found that many dancers consume less energy and nutrients than they need to support their health and performance.[9-14] In recent years, there has been a shift toward viewing dancers as artistic athletes, requiring the same attention to fueling for performance as has been prioritized in other sports. The stereotypical coffee and cigarette dancer diet of past eras may no longer be considered acceptable by most of the dance world, yet recent studies tell us that despite greater acknowledgment of the importance of nutrition, under-eating remains prevalent among dancers.[15-21]

When dancers consume fewer calories than needed to cover the energy cost of exercise, other activities of daily living, and normal body functioning, this creates an energy deficiency, also known as low energy availability (LEA). Low energy availability is of particular concern because it is the root cause of multiple serious health and performance consequences for dancers (as discussed in more detail below) and has a worryingly high prevalence among dancers. For instance, Civil and colleagues found that 66% of female pre-professional ballet students had sub-optimal energy intakes.[18] In a study with male and female dancers of various genres (mostly ballet), 57% of female dancers and 29% of male dancers had characteristics indicative of LEA.[19] Ninety-six percent of female college ballet dancers in a recent study had LEA.[20] Similar results were found in female breakdance, hip hop, and jazz dancers where only 4% had sufficient energy intakes.[21]

Female Athlete Triad

The Female Athlete Triad (Triad) is common among physically active girls and women and refers to three interrelated issues—energy availability, menstrual function, and bone health—each of which occurs on a spectrum as follows[22,23]:

- Energy availability—from optimal to LEA
- Menstrual function—from normal to amenorrhea
- Bone health—from optimal to osteoporosis

In Figure 2.1, the top image represents the healthy end of the Triad (which I have renamed the Dancer Triad and which illustrates the spectrum in girls/women and boys/men) where a dancer is fueling optimally. This means they have a healthy relationship with food and exercise and eat enough to support their training, daily activities, and their physical and mental health. Proper fueling helps the dancer to have normal hormone levels, regular periods, and optimal bone health. If the dancer eats less than is needed for health and performance (suboptimal fueling)—perhaps due to disordered eating, but not always—hormones, periods, and/or bone health may begin to be affected. In the middle portion of the spectrum, the dancer's health is impacted, but changes may be subclinical or less noticeable (e.g., lighter periods, reduced bone mineral density [BMD]) and are less severe than at the end of the continuum.

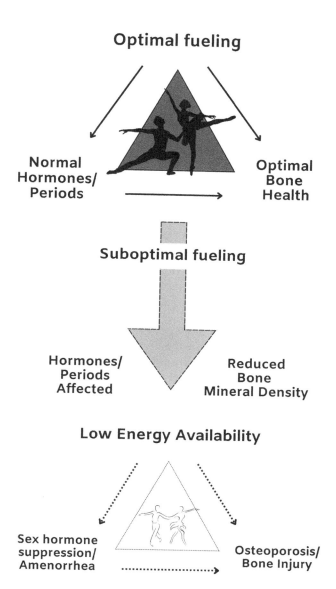

Figure 2.1 The Dancer Triad.

Created by the author (image credit © cundra703s-images and © oxygen-64 via Canva.com). Adapted from DeSouza et al., 2014[23] and Nattiv et al., 2021.[24]

When a dancer eats substantially below their needs for a more prolonged period, this results in LEA, which may be due to more severe disordered eating, an eating disorder, or other causes. This unhealthy end of the Triad spectrum is characterized by amenorrhea (i.e., functional hypothalamic amenorrhea) and osteoporosis.

The arrows in Figure 2.1 show the interrelated nature of the Triad components. Inadequate fueling directly impacts both bone health and hormones/periods, and hormonal/menstrual dysfunction also directly affects bone health.[23] The duration and severity of the energy deficiency will affect the outcomes. Some of these outcomes, such as diminished bone density, may be irreversible.[22]

The Triad won't present the same way in every dancer. A dancer may have disordered eating and stress fractures, but their menstrual cycle appears normal.[25] Two dancers may decrease their intake by the same amount, but only one stops menstruating. The exact threshold of LEA that leads to menstrual dysfunction is unknown and will vary by dancer. However, the greater the energy deficit, the more likely that there will be menstrual disturbances.[24]

Menstrual Periods—What's Normal, What's Not?

The belief that it's "normal" (and perhaps more convenient) for dancers not to menstruate due to their high levels of physical activity is a harmful myth I continue to hear perpetuated, even by physicians. However, as sports/dance endocrinologist Dr. Nicky Keay states, "All women of reproductive age, however much exercise is being undertaken, should have regular menstrual cycles, which is indicative of healthy hormones."[26] Unfortunately, menstrual dysfunction is prevalent among dancers.[18,19,27,28] Although there can be several potential causes of menstrual irregularities, under-fueling is often the culprit in dancers and athletes.

Amenorrhea—the absence of periods—should not be ignored or dismissed in dancers unless there is an explanation (e.g., pregnancy, breastfeeding, menopause, medications [including some contraceptives], etc.)[1] as both delayed menarche and amenorrhea lower BMD.[29] Dancers who do not get their first period by age 15 (primary amenorrhea) or after menarche do not get a period for three or more months (secondary amenorrhea) should be evaluated by a doctor,[1] ideally one who is familiar with the Triad.

What's "normal" in terms of period onset, frequency, duration, and flow will vary somewhat from dancer to dancer. According to the American College of Obstetricians and Gynecologists (ACOG), in addition to amenorrhea, menstrual abnormalities that warrant further evaluation include[30,31]:

- Periods that have not started within three years of breast budding
- Menstrual cycles shorter than 21 days or longer than 35 days in adults/45 days in adolescents (menstrual cycle length is measured from the first day of bleeding of one period to the first day of bleeding of the next period)

- Periods that last more than seven days
- Spotting or bleeding between periods
- Heavy flow requiring pad or tampon changes every one to two hours

In addition to addressing the menstrual abnormalities listed above, it's important for dancers to be aware of changes to their "normal" patterns (e.g., longer/shorter cycles, lighter/heavier bleeding), as this may be a sign of inadequate nutrition or other issues needing attention. Even subtle menstrual disturbances, which are difficult to detect and likely quite common in dancers, can negatively impact bone health.[32] In a study by De Souza and colleagues, daily hormone measurements confirmed a high prevalence of menstrual dysfunction in physically active women, including in women with menstrual cycles that appeared to be of normal length.[33] Therefore, having periods that seem "normal" does not necessarily indicate that a dancer is fueling adequately or that bone health is not being compromised.

Male Athlete Triad

The negative consequences of under-fueling on hormones and bone health are not just limited to girls/women. In 2021, the Female and Male Athlete Triad Coalition introduced a model for the Male Athlete Triad.[24] Adolescent and young adult male athletes in sports that require a lean physique, like dance, are most at risk.[34] The Male Athlete Triad also includes three interrelated areas (i.e., energy availability, reproductive function, bone health) which occur on a spectrum with some differences from the Female Athlete Triad.

In terms of energy availability, which goes from optimal to suboptimal to energy deficiency/LEA, it's not as clear in males how much of an energy deficit is needed to cause hormonal disruptions or impact bone health. However, it seems that a more severe energy deficiency, perhaps for a longer duration, is likely needed in males compared to females.[24] The hormonal health part of the Triad in males ranges from normal to suppression of reproductive hormones (e.g., testosterone) where libido and sperm quality and quantity may also be affected. The middle part of the spectrum is not as well defined but involves more subtle changes in the system that regulates the production of testosterone.[24] Bone health occurs on a continuum from optimal to reduced BMD and/or increased risk of bone injury to osteoporosis with or without bone injury.[24] Unfortunately, a bone stress injury may be one of the first noticeable signs of the Triad in males[34] because subtle changes in reproductive hormones may be harder to detect (vs. period changes in females).

Dance educators, staff, parents, and healthcare providers can help with early identification and intervention of the Triad in all dancers by being on the lookout for signs, symptoms, and risk factors, which may be subtle or overt (see the What to Screen For section). Dancers may have any or all the components of the Triad. If you observe that a dancer is exhibiting one aspect of the Triad, they should be evaluated for the others as well.[23,34] The goal is to intervene as early as possible to prevent progression to the end-points of the Triad spectrum.[23]

Relative Energy Deficiency in Sport (RED-S)

In 2014, the International Olympic Committee (IOC) introduced the term Relative Energy Deficiency in Sport (RED-S) as an expansion of the Female Athlete Triad to highlight that energy deficiency (i.e., too little intake *relative* to what is needed for activity and life) impacts all genders, not just females, and the consequences on health and performance extend far beyond just periods and bones.[5] The three interrelated conditions of the Triad are included within the RED-S concept. As in the Triad, insufficient energy intake is the root cause of the health and performance consequences of RED-S. Energy deficiency may be intentional or unintentional and related to disordered eating, an eating disorder, or other causes.[5] Dancers in all genres and at all levels from recreational to elite professional can be affected.

Health Consequences of RED-S

When your body doesn't get enough fuel to do everything it needs to, it con-serves energy to keep you alive. Body functions that are not vital for life (e.g., making reproductive hormones) may slow or shut down, which is necessary for survival but negatively affects health. RED-S can cause serious consequences in most body systems, including but not limited to those shown in Figure 2.2. The relationship between the various factors is more complex and interre-lated than depicted in the graphic. For example, under-fueling can lead to iron deficiency anemia and anemia may also lower appetite and therefore contribute to under-eating.[35] In addition, the impact of RED-S on the cardio-vascular system in females is at least in part related to low estrogen levels.[36] The main takeaway is that RED-S can have a profound impact on many aspects of dancers' physical and mental health.

As with the Triad, there is a lot of variability in how RED-S may affect dancers, and more research is needed to better understand how dancers of different genders, races, and ethnic backgrounds are impacted.[35] Examples of some of the health consequences that an under-fueled dancer may experi-ence are listed below. This list can also be used as a reminder of the warning signs and symptoms of RED-S that anyone who trains or cares for dancers should keep an eye out for. A dancer may have any or all of these, and they can occur in varying degrees of severity.

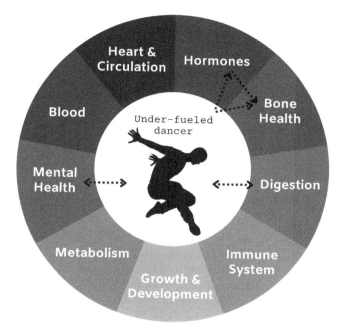

Figure 2.2 Health Consequences of Under-Fueling in Dancers.

Created by the author (image credit © geoimages via Canva.com). Adapted from Mountjoy et al., 2014.[5]

Hematological (blood and blood cells): Iron deficiency and anemia may develop in dancers—especially females—who are not eating enough.[35]

Cardiovascular (heart and blood vessels): Blood vessels may narrow and/or plaque may build up in arteries increasing the risk of heart disease.[35,36] Heart rate, blood pressure, and heart function may be affected, especially if a dancer has an eating disorder.[35] Dizziness and feeling lightheaded may also be symptoms of the cardiovascular impacts of RED-S.

Endocrine (hormones): Lower levels of reproductive hormones (e.g., estrogen, testosterone) contribute to menstrual dysfunction, low sex drive, poor bone health, and potential fertility issues.[23,34] Thyroid hormones, appetite hormones, growth hormone, and cortisol might also be affected.[35]

Bone health: As discussed in the Triad sections above, energy deficiency and hormone dysfunction can lead to lower bone density, an increased risk of stress fractures, and osteoporosis.

Gastrointestinal (digestion): Stomach aches, bloating, constipation, and feeling like "food is just sitting there" are common complaints from dancers who are under-fueling.[35] The bi-directional arrow in Figure 2.2 highlights that

RED-S may be the cause of digestive issues, and digestive issues also contribute to the development of RED-S.

Immune system: Decreased immune function may mean dancers have more frequent illnesses and infections,[5] and when they are sick, recovery may take longer.

Growth and development: Young dancers' height and weight may not increase as expected (e.g., the dancer "falls off" their usual growth chart curve) and unfortunately, catch-up growth is not always possible.[5,35] Pubertal development may also be delayed.

Metabolism: When faced with insufficient fuel, a dancer's metabolic rate will slow to conserve energy,[35] which is why RED-S does not always result in weight loss. Having a stable weight should not be viewed as a sign that a dancer is fueling optimally.

Mental health: Under-fueling can increase anxiety and depression and lower a dancer's ability to handle stress.[35] The double-headed arrow in Figure 2.2 highlights that psychological issues contribute to RED-S and vice versa. For example, negative energy balance is a risk factor for developing disordered eating/eating disorders, and disordered eating/eating disorders are major contributing factors to energy deficiency in dancers. In addition, depression and anxiety often decrease appetite and may lead to reduced intake.

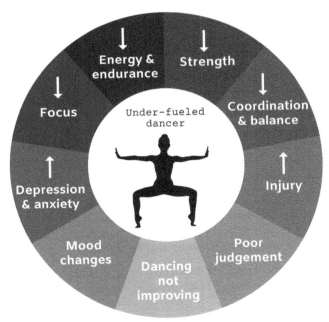

Figure 2.3 Performance Consequences of Under-Fueling in Dancers.

Created by the author (image credit © superuser1945s-images and © googledesignicons via Canva.com). Adapted from Mountjoy et al., 2014.[5]

Performance Consequences of RED-S

The effects of under-fueling on performance may be easier for parents, dance educators, and dancers to spot than some of the health consequences. The negative impacts on performance usually also resonate more with dancers. Struggling to focus during rehearsal or having an injury that keeps them out of dance can motivate a dancer to improve their eating habits once they understand the connection between nutrition and their dancing. The good news is that many of the health and performance effects of RED-S are reversible when caught and treated early.

As shown in Figure 2.3, a dancer who is not fueling optimally may experience:

- Difficulty focusing and concentrating, which may make it harder to learn combinations and choreography and lead to making more mistakes in classes and rehearsals
- Less energy, worse endurance, more fatigue
- Weakness, decreased strength
- Worse coordination and balance, slower reaction time[37,38]
- Frequent or slow-healing injuries
- Poor judgment—an undernourished brain is not a clear-thinking brain
- A lack of expected improvement in technique, strength, and/or artistry despite hard work and increased effort
- Irritability, depression, anxiety, isolation (psychological factors impact both health and performance)

There is substantial interplay between the various factors as well as between the health consequences and performance consequences. For example, increased fatigue and difficulty focusing can increase injury risk, and injury can cause or worsen psychological distress. Psychological and physical factors can both contribute to diminished progress in dancing.

Spotlight on Bone Health

Late childhood and the years around puberty are a critical time for bone building[39] with up to 90% of bone mass accrued by late adolescence.[40] Most dancers will attain their peak bone mass in their twenties with additional small increases possible in some bone sites until their early thirties.[40,41] Genetics play a significant role in bone health.[39] Although genetics can't be changed, several factors can be addressed to improve bone health, particularly nutritional factors.

Under-fueling can have damaging effects on a dancer's bones and is especially risky for pre-teen and adolescent dancers. If dancers don't consume enough calories and the necessary macro- and micro-nutrients to support healthy bone development during their peak bone-building years, the consequences may be irreversible. Even moderate energy deficits may suppress bone formation and keep adolescent dancers from reaching their full bone strength potential, which can occur even if periods appear normal.[22]

Delayed menarche impairs bone health,[42] and it is estimated that women with amenorrhea will lose 2–3% of their bone density per year.[43] So, ensuring that dancers' fueling practices support normal pubertal development and menstrual function is key. If menstrual abnormalities do occur, early treatment to restore periods is critical, which requires correcting nutrition deficiencies and often weight gain as well.[43,44]

A bone density test (e.g., dual-energy X-ray absorptiometry [DXA] scan) is recommended for dancers at risk for poor bone health including those with amenorrhea for six or more months.[45] A DXA should also be considered for dancers with other menstrual abnormalities (e.g., delayed menarche, infrequent periods), stress reactions/fractures, or indicators of poor nutrition such as current or past disordered eating/eating disorder, low weight, and/or recent weight loss.[23,34,45] Depending on a dancer's results and situation, a repeat DXA may be needed every one to two years.[23,34] Additional indications for bone density testing can be found in the Female and Male Athlete Triad Consensus Statements.[23,34]

In premenopausal females and males under 50, DXA results are reported as Z-scores[46] which compare the dancer's BMD at certain skeletal sites to age-, sex-, and often race- or ethnicity-matched controls.[45] Typically, a Z-score ≤ -2.0 is considered "below the expected range for age,"[46] but because dancers are expected to have higher bone density than the general population, a Z-score of < -1.0 is considered low BMD.[22,34] Osteoporosis is diagnosed if an adult dancer has a Z-score of ≤ -2.0 plus secondary risk factors for fracture (e.g., low estrogen, poor nutrition, prior fractures).[22,34] In children and adolescent dancers (ages 5–19), a diagnosis of osteoporosis requires low bone mass and a clinically significant fracture history.[46]

Although it's thought that sex differences (e.g., the protective effects of testosterone) make males less susceptible to the serious consequences of energy deficiency,[47] poor bone health is not only an issue among female dancers. A study of male and female adolescent elite ballet dancers found that over 30% had low BMD and of these dancers, nearly two-thirds were males.[48] In another study of professional ballet dancers, almost all the males and females had low BMD of the forearm, putting them at high risk for fractures.[28] Of note, although dance can be beneficial for improving bone mass in weight-bearing sites, the forearm doesn't get the same kind of impact in most dance genres, even in partnering lifts. According to the authors, this makes the forearm a more useful site to assess bone status in dancers because it will show impaired bone health before skeletal sites that receive more loading (e.g., hip), allowing for earlier intervention.[28]

Ensuring that dancers consume enough bone-building micronutrients such as calcium and vitamin D is necessary for the prevention and treatment of bone injuries. Exposure to sunlight is a major source of vitamin D, and there aren't many good food sources of this critical nutrient. Dancers who live in northern latitudes are at higher risk for having low levels, though vitamin D insufficiency and deficiency are concerns for all dancers considering how many hours they spend inside a studio. Dancers may benefit from having their vitamin D levels checked periodically to determine if a supplement is needed, and if so, the appropriate dosage. The Female and Male Athlete Triad Coalition recommends that blood levels of vitamin D be maintained at 32 ng/mL or above,[23,34] but dancers should consult with their medical team for individualized recommendations. More specific nutrition guidelines to support bone health are covered in Chapter 6.

Weight-bearing exercise (like dance) and strength training help in building and maintaining strong bones.[49] However, despite this potential benefit of dancing, dancers can still have poor bone health if they are under-fueling. Furthermore, adding additional exercise energy expenditure in an already undernourished dancer may be detrimental rather than beneficial. In particular, adding high-impact exercise in a dancer with low BMD is concerning as it may result in a fracture.[23]

Timing Matters—Within-Day Energy Deficiency

I frequently see dancers with eating patterns similar to Neil's habits described at the beginning of this chapter—skipping or skimping on breakfast, not eating much at lunch because of limited time, and then consuming the majority of their daily intake in the evening after they have finished most of their physical activity. Dancers may not realize that this lack of consistent fueling, especially during their busy dance day, can harm their health and performance.

Within-day energy deficiency refers to the times during the day that a dancer's energy intake is less than their energy expenditure. Experiencing these periods of negative energy balance may lead to undesirable consequences, even if total daily energy intake appears adequate. Within-day energy deficiency is associated with:

- Lower resting metabolic rate[50,51]
- Lower estrogen levels[50]
- Menstrual dysfunction[50]
- Increased injuries[52]
- Higher cortisol[50,51]
- Lower testosterone-to-cortisol ratio—a marker of catabolism and reduced ability to recover from exercise[51]
- Higher body fat percentage[53]

To improve performance, recovery, and health, dancers need to consume enough energy and nutrients overall and distribute their intake throughout the day to fuel their activity. Ideally, everyone involved in the training and care of dancers would support them in developing and maintaining optimal fueling practices (we'll discuss how in Acts II and III).

Contributing Factors

Andrew is a first-year dance major in a college conservatory program. He became vegan six months ago after watching a documentary on the harms of consuming animal products and reading social media posts recommending vegan diets for athletes. Several of his dance friends are also vegan. His current dance schedule is more intense than it was in high school. He lives in the dorms and has the college meal plan. Andrew is so tired in the morning that he often doesn't wake up early enough to get breakfast before class. He's starving by lunch, but by the time he walks to the cafeteria and gets through the line, he only has 15 minutes to eat before rehearsal. Andrew doesn't want to feel too full while dancing, so he just eats a few bites of lunch. There's usually at least one vegan option like pasta with vegetables offered for dinner. Sometimes the cafeteria has tofu available, but Andrew avoids it because he doesn't like its taste and he's heard soy causes cancer. Andrew rarely feels satisfied after meals. Many of his classmates buy food to supplement the meal plan, but finances are tight for Andrew's family, so he doesn't have money to purchase extra food. As the semester goes on, he notices he's always feeling fatigued and can't stop thinking about food. He becomes more anxious about his food choices, worrying that he won't make the "right" choice for his body or the environment.

As Andrew's story demonstrates, there are multiple factors that can contribute to dancers consuming less energy and/or nutrients than they need. Under-fueling is prevalent among dancers across genres and levels, and it may be unintentional or intentional. For example, a dancer may feel less hungry due to stress, anxiety, or increased training and may unconsciously eat less than usual or required. Or, when a dancer's activity level increases during the busy performance season, they may not realize they need extra fuel. Biological, psychological, or environmental issues might affect when, what, or how much a dancer eats. A dancer may also intentionally decrease what or how much they eat to lose weight or change their body. Or it may be a combination of any or all of these factors. Disordered eating and eating disorders are major contributors to inadequate fueling and will be discussed in detail in Chapter 3. Other common, often interrelated, causes of under-fueling in dancers include:

Diet vs. Dieting

The word "diet" has different definitions. Diet can refer to the food and beverages usually consumed or can mean an eating plan that restricts amounts, types of foods, or the way foods are prepared or consumed.[54] A diet may be followed for cultural, religious, or other personal reasons (e.g., kosher, halal, vegetarian diet). A diet may also be necessary for medical reasons like eliminating gluten if you have celiac disease. However, most restrictive dieting is unnecessary, such as when it is done to lose weight, change appearance, or "cleanse" or "detox." When discussing the harms of dieting, I am mostly referring to unnecessary restrictive diets.

Dieting is so normalized that we often don't recognize it as problematic. But dieting, which is prevalent both in our society and in the dance world, is neither a normal nor a healthy way of eating. As covered in Chapter 1, dieting harms dancers' physical and mental health and performance in a multitude of ways—it can lead to energy and nutrient deficiencies and is often the catalyst to developing an eating disorder. In fact, I consider dieting to be a form of disordered eating.

Because dancers are at high risk for eating disorders and under-fueling, I recommend that any dancer following a restricted diet speak with a dietitian, even if the diet is not for the purpose of weight loss. For example, although it is possible to have a healthy vegan or vegetarian diet, the motivation for following this type of diet should be explored, and dancers often need guidance to ensure they are fueling adequately. Even therapeutic diets should be recommended with extreme caution. I have had several dancer clients who were prescribed the low-FODMAP diet for irritable bowel syndrome (IBS) which precipitated their developing an eating disorder. Restrictive and hard-to-follow diets like this should be recommended as a last resort, only under the guidance of a dietitian, and with appropriate follow-up to help ensure that dancers are meeting their nutrition needs with the least restrictions possible and that the therapeutic diet is not contributing to disordered thoughts or behaviors.

Busy Schedules

Dancers' packed schedules can make eating enough a challenge. Juggling school, dance classes, rehearsals, work, physical therapy appointments, strength and conditioning sessions, and other obligations is not an easy feat. Dance schedules may allot 30 minutes for lunch, but it's not unusual for classes or rehearsals to run over, leaving the dancer with little time to use the restroom, change dance clothes and/or shoes, get their lunch, eat, digest, and be ready to dance again. Addressing these potential obstacles to fueling properly requires preparation and planning from dancers and their families (e.g., packing easy-to-eat/high-nutrient-density meals and snacks) and requires dance companies and schools to prioritize nutrition by scheduling adequate breaks for dancers to eat.

Access

Dancers come from varying socioeconomic backgrounds. Some are able to nourish their bodies without giving much thought to the cost of food. For others, financial constraints may impact their ability to meet their nutritional needs by limiting the types and/or quantity of food they can purchase. Additionally, a dancer's circumstances (e.g., if they have financial support from their family) and where a dancer lives (e.g., food deserts, expensive cities with a high cost of living) might affect what/how much they buy. These factors need to be considered and sensitively addressed when providing education and counseling to dancers.

Lack of Knowledge

Dancers can't nourish their bodies for optimal health and performance unless they know how to do so. Studies have found that knowledge about both nutrition[55-57] and the consequences of under-fueling[19,58] is often lacking in dancers. In my work with dancers, I frequently see knowledge deficits and confusion regarding necessary nutrients, their functions, good food sources, and the importance of meal timing as well as a lack of understanding about the harms of dieting and inadequate nutrition. Nutrition education is essential for dancers. In addition to learning how to meet their energy and nutrient needs, dancers benefit from being taught how to better match fueling to changing physical demands and when strategic eating is needed vs. relying on hunger cues. Dance educators, parents, and healthcare providers also need to know about these topics (see Chapter 6) so they can help dancers develop and maintain healthy habits.

Misinformation

Dancers, like the rest of us, are exposed to a lot of misinformation, especially on social media and the internet. Widespread inaccurate, misleading, and sometimes harmful claims go hand in hand with a lack of sound nutrition knowledge to contribute to confusion and food beliefs and behaviors that are not in dancers' best interest. In a recent study by Keay and colleagues, the main sources for nutrition information reported by pre-professional, professional, and advanced amateur dancers were the internet (61%), dietitian/nutritionist (32%), and friends or teachers at their school/company (29%).[19] I found similar results in a small informal survey that I did with pre-professional ballet dancers, where friend or family was the most common source of nutrition information reported by 53% of dancers, followed by the internet (50%), and healthcare provider (doctor, dietitian, etc.) (47%). Although it is encouraging that some dancers are getting nutrition information from qualified professionals (i.e., dietitian), the other popular sources are concerning, especially considering that about 40% of the dancers in the Keay study were advised by teachers/other dancers to exclude certain foods—most frequently carbohydrates.[19]

Often willing to do whatever it takes to achieve their goals, dancers are vulnerable to diets and products that purport to aid in weight loss or fat-burning as well as those that claim to improve energy or performance. They are also susceptible to following advice and recommendations that come from teachers, dancers, influencers, and other people they admire and trust. Unfortunately, as in the carbohydrate example above, recommendations from unqualified sources are often counterproductive to health and performance.

Dancers need to learn how to critically evaluate nutrition information. How can they tell if a source is credible? What qualifications or training should people that they seek advice from have? Even if the person has the recommended credentials, how will the dancer know if the advice is right for them? Chapter 6 provides guidance to discern nutrition fact from fiction and to help dancers figure out if a diet or way of eating is beneficial for their health and well-being. The Appendix contains recommendations to assist in finding qualified healthcare professionals.

Empty Tank of Artistry

Thus far, I've focused on the ways poor fueling can affect dancers' health and performance. It's also important to mention how being in a nutritionally depleted state can diminish artistry. How can a dancer be fully present and reach their full potential when their brain and body aren't functioning optimally? Dieting, disordered eating, and eating disorders—common contributors to under-fueling—drain a dancer physically and mentally, leaving little energy and space for creativity. Regardless of the cause, under-fueling is a source of stress for the mind and body that can lessen the fulfillment and joy that dancers get from their art and dim the unique light that each dancer brings to the art form.

Screening and Treatment
It Will Take All of Us

The health and performance consequences of under-fueling can be serious, and some outcomes, such as reduced bone density, may be irreversible. Children and adolescents are particularly vulnerable to the effects of inadequate nutrition given the increased energy and nutrient needs of growth and development. Everyone who trains and cares for dancers should be aware of the signs and symptoms of the Triad, RED-S, and other indicators that a dancer may be under-fueling. We all have a valuable role to play in prevention, early identification, and prompt intervention when issues arise. The sooner nutrition deficiencies are addressed, the less likely that the dancer will suffer lasting damage.

Elements of Screening

Screening is a key part of prevention and early identification that helps catch potential concerns before they develop into more serious issues. Anyone who works with dancers can screen, but physical therapists, athletic trainers, primary care physicians, and other healthcare providers are in a particularly good position to identify dancers at risk for or already experiencing the impacts of under-fueling. Screening questions can be incorporated into intake forms with additional monitoring at follow-up visits. It's important to note that information collected in screenings is protected health information and needs to be kept confidential according to rules that safeguard this type of sensitive data. Dancers (and/or parents/guardians in the case of minors) should know how information from screenings will be used and provide consent if it will be shared.

Guidelines for screening are discussed below. The presence of any of the listed risk factors, signs, or symptoms indicates the need for further assessment. Before screening a dancer, it's necessary to have a plan in place for next steps (e.g., communicating findings with the dancer, referring to other providers, involving parents of young dancers).

When to screen: Dancers should be screened at their annual physical, pre-season medical exam, and any time an issue related to under-fueling is present, including injury, menstrual irregularity, disordered eating, or weight loss.[5,22,34]

What to screen for: Energy deficiency is the cause of the Triad and RED-S, so assessing how dancers' intake compares with their needs is essential. Unfortunately, calculating energy availability is difficult, time-consuming, and estimates are often inaccurate. The detailed tracking of food and exercise required to measure energy availability may increase food/calorie obsession and be triggering for dancers with disordered eating/eating disorders. In addition, evaluating a few days of energy intake and expenditure does not provide a full picture of a dancer's eating patterns and may not reveal areas of concern.

There are still a lot of unknowns about how the duration, timing, and severity of an energy deficiency affects outcomes. The consequences of LEA will also vary depending on each dancer's genetics and other individual factors, so the same energy deficit may cause amenorrhea and stress fractures in one dancer and no perceptible signs in another. A detailed nutrition assessment done by a dietitian with experience in RED-S, eating disorders, and dance is the best way to evaluate the adequacy of a dancer's intake.

Given the complications with calculating energy availability, it's helpful to ask dancers about factors associated with under-fueling such as:

- **Weight concerns**: Do they worry about their weight? Are they trying to gain or lose weight? Do they feel pressure to change their body size/shape? Have they heard any negative comments about their weight/shape?[23,34]
- **Restrictive eating**: Are there any foods or food groups they avoid or limit (e.g., dairy, gluten)? Are they currently following any type of diet (e.g., vegetarian, calorie-restricted)? Have they been on any diets previously?[23,34]

- **Excessive or compulsive exercise**: Have they increased their exercise volume or intensity? If so, are they eating more? What are their motivations for exercise (e.g., to control weight, get stronger, manage stress)? How do they feel if they miss a planned workout?
- **Body image dissatisfaction**: How do they feel about their body? Are they satisfied with their body size/shape?
- **Disordered eating/eating disorders**: Do they currently have or have they ever had disordered eating or an eating disorder?[23,34]

In addition, dancers should be screened for indicators of LEA and signs and symptoms of the Triad and RED-S, shown in Table 2.2. Low weight, weight loss, and lack of expected growth and development in dancers are red flags that warrant prompt attention. However, because under-fueling slows metabolism, a stable or "normal" weight does not guarantee that a dancer is fueling adequately. Similarly, seemingly normal periods do not necessarily mean that a dancer is eating enough or at a weight that best supports their physical and mental health. It is important to ask dancers about their use of birth control pills or other hormonal contraceptives which may mask menstrual dysfunction. Blood tests may be helpful to assess additional indicators of LEA such as reproductive hormone abnormalities and thyroid function.[59]

Screening tools: Healthcare providers and dance practitioners may find it helpful to incorporate existing screening tools into their practice. The most suitable choice will depend on your role and the setting in which you work with dancers.

Table 2.2 Warning Signs and Symptoms of Under-Fueling in Dancers

Hormonal dysfunction: Delayed menarche, history of/current menstrual abnormalities, lower libido, less frequent shaving of facial hair and/or absence of/fewer morning erections (in post-pubertal males)
Weight: Low-weight, weight loss, lack of expected weight gain/growth/development in children and adolescents
Injuries: Current/past stress fractures or other bone injury, recurring or slow-healing injuries
Signs and symptoms of eating disorders
Low bone density
Frequent or prolonged illnesses
Digestive issues
Mood changes
Fatigue
Impaired performance

Adapted from DeSouza et al., 2014[23]; Fredericson et al., 2021[34]; and Mountjoy et al., 2014.[5]

The Female and Male Athlete Triad Coalition and IOC authors have created tools to assist in screening for the Triad and RED-S respectively, as well as to help with decisions about whether a dancer may need to decrease, modify, or stop training and performing.[23,34,60] Clinical judgment that takes a dancer's specific situation into account should guide decisions regarding removal from dance (more on this in Chapter 3). Links for various screening tools are provided in the Appendix.

Treatment for Under-Fueling

The primary goal of screening is to identify possible issues and refer the dancer to specialized providers as soon as possible for further evaluation and management. A multidisciplinary approach to treatment is often needed to treat the consequences of under-fueling and address contributing factors. Team members may include a physician, dietitian, psychotherapist, physical therapist, and/or psychiatrist.

Because LEA is the underlying cause of the Triad and RED-S, correcting the energy deficiency needs to be the initial focus of treatment. Nutrition counseling with a dietitian can help improve the adequacy of a dancer's diet, which includes addressing any macro- or micro-nutrient deficiencies. A dietitian can also help the dancer create an eating plan that provides consistent fueling throughout the day. Gradual increases in intake are usually recommended, but pacing should not be too slow because allowing dancers, particularly young dancers, to remain in a state of LEA for long periods may have irreversible consequences for bone health. In some cases, it may be necessary for the dancer to decrease energy expenditure as well.

If lack of knowledge, misinformation, or hectic schedules are the reasons for under-fueling, nutrition counseling may be sufficient to improve the dancer's intake. When other factors such as disordered eating/eating disorders are present, more extensive care from a multidisciplinary team is needed. Anyone working with dancers should be familiar with eating disorders, so they know when to refer to a specialist and have a list of providers to refer to.

Increasing energy availability is necessary to correct hormonal/menstrual dysfunction and improve bone health. As mentioned earlier, weight gain is often needed as well.[23,45] Sometimes only small amounts of weight gain will be needed, but the degree of weight restoration required is highly individual. Ultimately, it is the dancer's body that determines where it functions optimally—not the dancer's school, company, parent, or even their medical providers.

Under-fueling doesn't immediately cause a reduction in bone density, and improvements in fueling won't automatically correct hormones or restore bones to full health. Energy intake can typically be improved in days to weeks, followed by weight increases over weeks to months.[23] Restoration of normal menstrual/hormonal function will likely take several months, though it could take a year or more.[23] Bone density is the slowest to recover—it may take years and full recovery may not be possible in some cases.[23] Although hormonal/menstrual dysfunction usually responds to improved nutrition, which both in turn help improve bone health, medication management may be recommended for some dancers who don't respond to treatment after one year.[23,34] Additional interventions are especially important to consider in young dancers because failure to achieve their full bone mass potential in their critical bone-building years could have devastating consequences.[23]

Oral contraceptive pills are not recommended for the purpose of regaining menses or improving bone health[45] (though there are other reasons a dancer may choose to take them). Oral contraceptive pills neither "jump start" periods nor do they protect bones, though unfortunately they continue to be prescribed for these reasons.[61] Dancers should know that oral contraceptives cause withdrawal bleeding, which is not the same thing as getting a period naturally.[62] This effect can give a false sense of security and preclude the use of restoration of natural periods as an indicator of improved hormonal function.[23,45]

In some cases, short-term transdermal estradiol therapy (aka the estrogen patch) given with cyclic oral progesterone may be considered to protect the bones of dancers who do not respond to nutritional and psychological treatment and/or reduced exercise.[45] This use is meant as an adjunct to, not a substitute for, the primary goal of adequate nutrition and weight restoration.[61,63] The Female and Male Athlete Triad Consensus Statements[23,34] and the Endocrine Society's Functional Hypothalamic Amenorrhea Practice Guideline[45] provide additional details on pharmacological interventions and indications for their use.

Treatment recommendations need to consider each dancer's unique needs and preferences and be tailored to their specific circumstances. Ideally, prevention efforts help dancers avoid the serious health and performance consequences of under-fueling so that treatment is not needed. The dancer and the dance world have much to gain from prioritizing optimal fueling. A well-nourished dancer is a healthier, happier dancer who will feel better, perform better, be less likely to get injured, and be more likely to reach their full potential as an artist and a human.

Main Pointes

- Under-fueling is prevalent in dancers and has serious consequences for their health and performance.
- Children and adolescents are particularly vulnerable to the effects of inadequate nutrition.
- Energy deficiency is the underlying cause of the Triad and RED-S; therefore, ensuring dancers are consuming enough energy and nutrients needs to be the focus of prevention and treatment.
- Common contributing factors to under-fueling in dancers include disordered eating, eating disorders, dieting, schedules, access, lack of knowledge, and misinformation.

- Many of the effects of under-fueling get better with improved nutrition, but negative impacts on bone health may be irreversible.
- The belief that it's "normal" for dancers not to menstruate due to their high levels of physical activity is a harmful myth.
- Oral contraceptive pills should not be used for the purpose of restoring periods or improving bone health.
- Anyone who trains or cares for dancers can improve dancers' health and performance by helping to create an environment that encourages and supports optimal fueling.
- Dance educators/staff, parents, and healthcare providers should be aware of the risk factors, signs, and symptoms of under-fueling. We all have a key role to play in prevention, early identification, and timely treatment.

Notes

Think about dancers you train or care for. What risk factors for under-fueling have you noticed? What signs and symptoms of the Triad or RED-S have you observed?

What obstacles to optimal fueling in dancers have you encountered? What might help to reduce these barriers?

References

1. American College of Obstetricians and Gynecologists (ACOG). Amenorrhea: Absence of periods. October 2020. Accessed November 6, 2022. https://www.acog.org/womens-health/faqs/amenorrhea-absence-of-periods
2. Harvard Health Publishing Harvard Medical School. Medical dictionary of health terms. December 13, 2011. Accessed November 6, 2022. https://www.health.harvard.edu/a-through-c#B-terms
3. Ma S-Y (Richard). Bone mineral density. Encyclopædia Britannica. Accessed November 6, 2022. https://www.britannica.com/science/bone-mineral-density
4. The Female and Male Athlete Triad Coalition. What is energy deficiency/Low EA? Accessed November 6, 2022. https://femaleandmaleathletetriad.org/athletes/what-is-energy-deficiency-energy-availability/
5. Mountjoy M, Sundgot-Borgen J, Burke L, et al. The IOC consensus statement: Beyond the Female Athlete Triad–Relative Energy Deficiency in Sport (RED-S). *Br J Sports Med.* 2014;48(7):491–497. doi:10.1136/bjsports-2014-093502
6. Cleveland Clinic. Q&A: Is hypothalamic amenorrhea to blame for your missed periods? September 4, 2019. Accessed November 6, 2022. https://health.clevelandclinic.org/q-and-a-is-hypothalamic-amenorrhea-to-blame-for-your-missed-periods/
7. National Institutes of Health. Osteoporosis overview. Accessed November 6, 2022. https://www.bones.nih.gov/health-info/bone/osteoporosis/overview
8. Bone Health & Osteoporosis Foundation. Peak bone mass. Accessed November 6, 2022. https://www.bonehealthandosteoporosis.org/preventing-fractures/nutrition-for-bone-health/peak-bone-mass/
9. Benson J, Gillien DM, Bourdet K, Loosli AR. Inadequate nutrition and chronic calorie restriction in adolescent ballerinas. *Phys Sportsmed.* 1985;13(10):79–90. doi:10.1080/00913847.1985.11708902

10. Dahlström M, Jansson E, Nordevang E, Kaijser L. Discrepancy between estimated energy intake and requirement in female dancers. *Clin Physiol.* 1990;10(1):11–25. doi:10.1111/j.1475-097x.1990.tb00080.x

11. Hirsch N, Eisenmann J, Moore S, Winnail S, Stalder M. Energy balance and physical activity patterns in university ballet dancers. *J Dance Med Sci.* 2003;7:73–79.

12. Bonbright JM. The nutritional status of female ballet dancers 15–18 years of age. *Dance Res J.* 1989;21(2):9–14. doi:10.2307/1478626

13. Kostrzewa-Tarnowska A, Jeszko J. Energy balance and body composition factors in adolescent ballet school students. *Pol J Food Nutr Sci.* 2003;53(3):71–75.

14. Doyle-Lucas AF, Akers JD, Davy BM. Energetic efficiency, menstrual irregularity, and bone mineral density in elite professional female ballet dancers. *J Dance Med Sci.* 2010;14(4):146–154.

15. Beck KL, Mitchell S, Foskett A, Conlon CA, von Hurst PR. Dietary intake, anthropometric characteristics, and iron and vitamin D status of female adolescent ballet dancers living in New Zealand. *Int J Sport Nutr Exerc Metab.* 2015;25(4):335–343. doi:10.1123/ijsnem.2014-0089

16. Robbeson JG, Kruger HS, Wright HH. Disordered eating behavior, body image, and energy status of female student dancers. *Int J Sport Nutr Exerc Metab.* 2015;25(4):344–352. doi:10.1123/ijsnem.2013-0161

17. Brown MA, Howatson G, Quin E, Redding E, Stevenson EJ. Energy intake and energy expenditure of pre-professional female contemporary dancers. *PLoS ONE.* 2017;12(2):e0171998. doi:10.1371/journal.pone.0171998

18. Civil R, Lamb A, Loosmore D, et al. Assessment of dietary intake, energy status, and factors associated with RED-S in vocational female ballet students. *Front Nutr.* 2018;5:136. doi:10.3389/fnut.2018.00136

19. Keay N, Overseas A, Francis G. Indicators and correlates of low energy availability in male and female dancers. *BMJ Open Sport Exerc Med.* 2020;6(1):e000906. doi:10.1136/bmjsem-2020-000906

20. Torres-McGehee TM, Emerson DM, Pritchett K, Moore EM, Smith AB, Uriegas NA. Energy availability with or without eating disorder risk in collegiate female athletes and performing artists. *J Athl Train.* December 22, 2020. doi:10.4085/JAT0502-20

21. Prus D, Mijatovic D, Hadzic V, et al. (Low) energy availability and its association with injury occurrence in competitive dance: Cross-sectional analysis in female dancers. *Medicina (Kaunas).* 2022;58(7). doi:10.3390/medicina58070853

22. Nattiv A, Loucks AB, Manore MM, et al. American college of sports medicine position stand. The female athlete triad. *Med Sci Sports Exerc.* 2007;39(10):1867–1882. doi:10.1249/mss.0b013e318149f111

23. De Souza MJ, Nattiv A, Joy E, et al. 2014 Female athlete triad coalition consensus statement on treatment and return to play of the female athlete triad. 1st International Conference held in San Francisco, California, May 2012 and 2nd International Conference held in Indianapolis, Indiana, May 2013. *Br J Sports Med.* 2014;48(4):289. doi:10.1136/bjsports-2013-093218

24. Nattiv A, De Souza MJ, Koltun KJ, et al. The male athlete triad—A consensus statement from the female and male athlete triad coalition part 1: Definition and scientific basis. *Clin J Sport Med.* 2021;31(4):335–348. doi:10.1097/JSM.0000000000000946

25. Cobb KL, Bachrach LK, Greendale G, et al. Disordered eating, menstrual irregularity, and bone mineral density in female runners. *Med Sci Sports Exerc.* 2003;35(5):711–719. doi:10.1249/01.MSS.0000064935.68277.E7

26. Keay N. Raising awareness of RED-S in male and female athletes and dancers. Blog British Journal of Sports Medicine. October 30, 2018. Accessed October 13, 2022. https://blogs.bmj.com/bjsm/2018/10/30/raising-awareness-of-red-s-in-male-and-female-athletes-and-dancers/

27. Hincapié CA, Cassidy JD. Disordered eating, menstrual disturbances, and low bone mineral density in dancers: A systematic review. *Arch Phys Med Rehabil.* 2010;91(11):1777–1789.e1. doi:10.1016/j.apmr.2010.07.230

28. Gorwa J, Zieliński J, Wolański W, et al. Decreased bone mineral density in forearm vs loaded skeletal sites in professional ballet dancers. *Med Probl Perform Art.* 2019;34(1):25–32. doi:10.21091/mppa.2019.1006

29. Hewett E, Tufano J. Bone health in female ballet dancers: A review. *Eur J Sport Studies.* 2015;3(2).

30. American College of Obstetricians and Gynecologists Committee on Adolescent Health Care. ACOG Committee Opinion No. 651: Menstruation in girls and adolescents: Using the menstrual cycle as a vital sign. *Obstet Gynecol.* 2015;126(6):e143–6. doi:10.1097/AOG.0000000000001215

31. American College of Obstetricians and Gynecologists. Abnormal uterine bleeding. ACOG. December 2021. Accessed October 14, 2022. https://www.acog.org/womens-health/faqs/abnormal-uterine-bleeding

32. Li D, Hitchcock CL, Barr SI, Yu T, Prior JC. Negative spinal bone mineral density changes and subclinical ovulatory disturbances–Prospective data in healthy premenopausal women with regular menstrual cycles. *Epidemiol Rev.* 2014;36:137–147. doi:10.1093/epirev/mxt012

33. De Souza MJ, Toombs RJ, Scheid JL, O'Donnell E, West SL, Williams NI. High prevalence of subtle and severe menstrual disturbances in exercising women: Confirmation using daily hormone measures. *Hum Reprod.* 2010;25(2):491–503. doi:10.1093/humrep/dep411

34. Fredericson M, Kussman A, Misra M, et al. The male athlete triad-A consensus statement from the Female and Male Athlete Triad Coalition Part II: Diagnosis, treatment, and return-to-play. *Clin J Sport Med.* 2021;31(4):349–366. doi:10.1097/JSM.0000000000000948

35. Mountjoy M, Sundgot-Borgen JK, Burke LM, et al. IOC consensus statement on relative energy deficiency in sport (RED-S): 2018 update. *Br J Sports Med.* 2018;52(11):687–697. doi:10.1136/bjsports-2018-099193

36. O'Donnell E, Goodman JM, Harvey PJ. Clinical review: Cardiovascular consequences of ovarian disruption: A focus on functional hypothalamic amenorrhea in physically active women. *J Clin Endocrinol Metab.* 2011;96(12):3638–3648. doi:10.1210/jc.2011-1223

37. Keay N. Hormones and dance performance. *One Dance UK Information Sheet.*

38. Tornberg ÅB, Melin A, Koivula FM, et al. Reduced neuromuscular performance in amenorrheic elite endurance athletes. *Med Sci Sports Exerc.* 2017;49(12):2478–2485. doi:10.1249/MSS.0000000000001383

39. Weaver CM, Gordon CM, Janz KF, et al. The National Osteoporosis Foundation's position statement on peak bone mass development and lifestyle factors: A systematic review and implementation recommendations. *Osteoporos Int.* 2016;27(4):1281–1386. doi:10.1007/s00198-015-3440-3

40. Henry YM, Fatayerji D, Eastell R. Attainment of peak bone mass at the lumbar spine, femoral neck and radius in men and women: Relative contributions of bone size and volumetric bone mineral density. *Osteoporos Int.* 2004;15(4):263–273. doi:10.1007/s00198-003-1542-9

41. Baxter-Jones ADG, Faulkner RA, Forwood MR, Mirwald RL, Bailey DA. Bone mineral accrual from 8 to 30 years of age: An estimation of peak bone mass. *J Bone Miner Res.* 2011;26(8):1729–1739. doi:10.1002/jbmr.412

42. Burckhardt P, Wynn E, Krieg M-A, Bagutti C, Faouzi M. The effects of nutrition, puberty and dancing on bone density in adolescent ballet dancers. *J Dance Med Sci.* 2011;15(2):51–60.

43. Miller KK, Lee EE, Lawson EA, et al. Determinants of skeletal loss and recovery in anorexia nervosa. *J Clin Endocrinol Metab.* 2006;91(8):2931–2937. doi:10.1210/jc.2005-2818

44. Misra M, Prabhakaran R, Miller KK, et al. Weight gain and restoration of menses as predictors of bone mineral density change in adolescent girls with anorexia nervosa-1. *J Clin Endocrinol Metab.* 2008;93(4):1231–1237. doi:10.1210/jc.2007-1434

45. Gordon CM, Ackerman KE, Berga SL, et al. Functional hypothalamic amenorrhea: An endocrine society clinical practice guideline. *J Clin Endocrinol Metab.* 2017;102(5):1413–1439. doi:10.1210/jc.2017-00131

46. Lewiecki EM, Gordon CM, Baim S, et al. Special report on the 2007 adult and pediatric Position Development Conferences of the International Society for Clinical Densitometry. *Osteoporos Int.* 2008;19(10):1369–1378. doi:10.1007/s00198-008-0689-9

47. De Souza MJ, Williams NI, Nattiv A, et al. Misunderstanding the female athlete triad: Refuting the IOC consensus statement on Relative Energy Deficiency in Sport (RED-S). *Br J Sports Med.* 2014;48(20):1461–1465. doi:10.1136/bjsports-2014-093958

48. Wielandt T, van den Wyngaert T, Uijttewaal JR, Huyghe I, Maes M, Stassijns G. Bone mineral density in adolescent elite ballet dancers. *J Sports Med Phys Fitness.* 2019;59(9):1564–1570. doi:10.23736/S0022-4707.19.09700-7

49. The Female and Male Athlete Triad Coalition. Your bone health. Accessed November 6, 2022. https://femaleandmaleathletetriad.org/athletes/your-bone-health/

50. Fahrenholtz IL, Sjödin A, Benardot D, et al. Within-day energy deficiency and reproductive function in female endurance athletes. *Scand J Med Sci Sports.* 2018;28(3):1139–1146. doi:10.1111/sms.13030

51. Torstveit MK, Fahrenholtz I, Stenqvist TB, Sylta Ø, Melin A. Within-day energy deficiency and metabolic perturbation in male endurance athletes. *Int J Sport Nutr Exerc Metab.* 2018;28(4):419–427. doi:10.1123/ijsnem.2017-0337

52. Harrison E. Within-day energy balance and the relationship to injury rates in pre-professional ballet dancers. Thesis. Georgia State University; 2009. doi:10.57709/1062564

53. Deutz RC, Benardot D, Martin DE, Cody MM. Relationship between energy deficits and body composition in elite female gymnasts and runners. *Med Sci Sports Exerc.* 2000;32(3):659–668. doi:10.1097/00005768-200003000-00017

54. Cambridge Dictionary. Diet. Accessed November 6, 2022. https://dictionary.cambridge.org/us/dictionary/english/diet

55. Wyon MA, Hutchings KM, Wells A, Nevill AM. Body mass index, nutritional knowledge, and eating behaviors in elite student and professional ballet dancers. *Clin J Sport Med.* 2014;24(5):390–396. doi:10.1097/JSM.0000000000000054

56. Hanna K, Hanley A, Huddy A, McDonald M, Willer F. Physical activity participation and nutrition and physical activity knowledge in university dance students. *Med Probl Perform Art.* 2017;32(1):1–7. doi:10.21091/mppa.2017.1001

57. Mathisen TF, Sundgot-Borgen C, Anstensrud B, Sundgot-Borgen J. Intervention in professional dance students to increase mental health- and nutrition literacy: A controlled trial with follow up. *Front Sports Act Living.* 2022;4:727048. doi:10.3389/fspor.2022.727048

58. Tosi M, Maslyanskaya S, Dodson NA, Coupey SM. The female athlete triad: A comparison of knowledge and risk in adolescent and young adult figure skaters, dancers, and runners. *J Pediatr Adolesc Gynecol.* 2019;32(2):165–169. doi:10.1016/j.jpag.2018.10.007
59. Heikura IA, Uusitalo ALT, Stellingwerff T, Bergland D, Mero AA, Burke LM. Low energy availability is difficult to assess but outcomes have large impact on bone injury rates in elite distance athletes. *Int J Sport Nutr Exerc Metab.* 2018;28(4):403–411. doi:10.1123/ijsnem.2017-0313
60. Relative Energy Deficiency in Sport (RED-S). *Br J Sports Med.* 2015;49(7):421–423. doi:10.1136/bjsports-2014-094559
61. Gaudiani JL. *Sick Enough.* 1st ed. Routledge; 2018:276.
62. The Female and Male Athlete Triad Coalition. Myths vs. truths. Accessed November 6, 2022. https://femaleandmaleathletetriad.org/myths-truths/
63. British Journal of Sports Medicine. Female athlete hormone health 2022—NICE guideline update. May 18, 2022. Accessed November 6, 2022. https://blogs.bmj.com/bjsm/2022/05/18/female-athlete-hormone-health-2022-nice-guideline-update/

3   Eating Disorders and Disordered Eating in Dancers

[I]t's very hard to get over something when it is accepted.
~Female athlete [i]

What Are Eating Disorders?

Eating disorders are complex bio-psycho-social conditions that involve unhealthy feelings, beliefs, and behaviors around food, weight, body, and/or exercise. They are mental illnesses that cause significant emotional distress and physical health problems and are potentially life-threatening. There is no one cause of an eating disorder, but rather multiple genetic, psychological, and environmental factors that may contribute to developing one. Eating disorders have the second highest mortality rate of all mental health conditions following substance use disorders (primarily opioid use). [1]

The first time I remember thinking about the seriousness of eating disorders was in 1997 when Boston Ballet dancer Heidi Guenther died from complications of an eating disorder at age 22. Her story put a spotlight on eating disorders within the world of ballet. News stories focused on her low weight at the time of her death and how her drastic weight loss began after she was told to lose weight by the assistant artistic director of her ballet company. [2] Her death was tragic, not only because the world lost a young, talented dancer from a preventable and treatable condition, but also because her death wasn't the tipping point for accountability and meaningful change in the dance world. Instead, factors that undoubtedly contributed to the development of her eating disorder have been largely dismissed as "just how things are in ballet."

Heidi Guenther's death brought attention to many of the problematic issues in the dance world that needed to (and sadly 25 years later still need to) be addressed. The coverage of her story also reinforced a stereotype of what an eating disorder looks like in dance—young, female, White, visibly underweight. This harmful stereotype, which persists today, is not only

---

i Reprinted with permission from Arthur-Cameselle JN, Quatromoni PA. A Qualitative Analysis of Female Collegiate Athletes' Eating Disorder Recovery Experiences. *The Sport Psychologist.* 2014;28(4):334–346. doi:10.1123/tsp.2013-0079

DOI: 10.4324/9781003366171-4

inaccurate, but also a barrier to identification and treatment for all those who do not fit the narrow description. Eating disorders don't discriminate. They affect all ages, genders, ethnicities, races, sexual orientations, socio-economic groups, and body weights, sizes, and shapes in the dance world and beyond.

What examples come to mind when you think about stories of eating disorders you've seen covered in the media? Often, they are stories like Heidi's with obvious and expected warning signs (e.g., very low weight) and tragic outcomes. An unintended consequence of highlighting these cases is that it leads to others dismissing their own issues as "not that bad" in comparison. Many of my clients feel that they don't need or deserve help because they don't meet certain criteria they deem necessary to qualify as sick enough (abnormal labs, being underweight, needing hospitalization, etc.). Some, especially those prone to perfectionistic or black-and-white thinking, criticize themselves for being a failure ("I can't even be good at having an eating disorder") because their suffering is seemingly less severe or less visible.

Any dancer, any person, whose relationship with food, weight, exercise, or body image is negatively impacting their physical, emotional, or mental health in any way deserves help. There are substantial benefits to intervening early, long before the dancer may feel things are bad enough to warrant seeking help. The sooner the treatment, the better the chance of full recovery and the less likely there will be irreversible damage (e.g., to bone health or fertility). Everyone involved in the training and care of dancers has a critical role to play in the prevention and early intervention of eating disorders in dancers.

Disordered Eating vs. Eating Disorders

The terms "eating disorder" and "disordered eating" are often used interchangeably, and although related, they are not the same. You can think of these conditions as occurring on a spectrum as depicted in Figure 3.1.

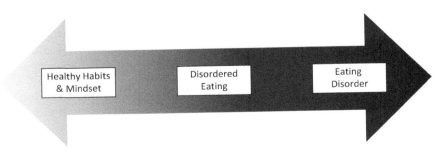

Figure 3.1 Eating Disorder Spectrum.

Healthy eating habits and a healthy relationship with food, body, and exercise are on one end, moving into disordered eating, and then eating disorders on the other end. Disordered eating can involve the same or similar behaviors as an eating disorder (e.g., restricting food intake, compensatory exercise, purging), but the behaviors don't happen as frequently or the consequences aren't as severe—yet.

Disordered eating frequently leads to an eating disorder; therefore, intervening early is crucial. In addition, dancers may move back and forth on the continuum between disordered eating and an eating disorder. When seeking help, dancers might encounter practitioners who say they work with clients with disordered eating but not eating disorders. Considering the fine, and at times indistinguishable, line separating disordered eating and eating disorders and that these behaviors are rarely static, I recommend dancers seek help from providers with expertise in treating eating disorders—even if the dancer isn't yet at that point on the spectrum. My hope is that we can all help dancers move toward and stay on the healthy part of the spectrum.

Eating Disorders Are Much Too Common

A recent review study on eating disorders in dancers, which included students and professionals and ballet along with other dance genres, found that dancers had a three times higher risk of having an eating disorder than non-dancers.[3] Eating disorder not otherwise specified (EDNOS)* was the most common eating disorder in dancers. Most of the studies included in this review were on ballet dancers, so researchers looked at ballet dancers separately. Compared to the prevalence of eating disorders found in the full group with various dance styles represented, ballet dancers had higher rates of anorexia nervosa, EDNOS, and eating disorders overall (though not bulimia nervosa).[3] An older study found that 83% of female ballet dancers had an eating disorder in their lifetime.[4] This number may seem shocking, but it's not that surprising when we consider all of the risk factors that exist in ballet.

Let's look at some research on two major contributing factors in eating disorder development—body dissatisfaction and unhealthy weight control behaviors. As discussed in Chapter 1, body image dissatisfaction and the use of harmful dieting practices are common among dancers across different genres. One study of 13–18-year-old female ballet students from competitive national schools as well as presumably less competitive regional and local studios found that about 60–70% wanted to lose weight (percent varies based on type of school—i.e., national vs. regional vs. local). Twenty-five to 40% of the adolescent dancers reported a history of fasting. The participants also reported other disordered behaviors such as compulsive exercise, vomiting, and laxative use.[5] It would be beneficial to research the prevalence of a broader range of disordered eating behaviors in dancers (e.g., various methods of food restriction, compensatory exercise and eating habits, rigid food rules, etc.).

Dancers frequently engage in these problematic practices, but because they are so normalized in our society, they are not named or viewed as disordered.

Most of the existing research on eating disorders in dancers is on female, predominantly White ballet dancers from companies, pre-professional programs, or other elite schools. However, a higher risk of eating disorders is not isolated to this genre or training setting. An increased risk for eating disorders and disordered eating has also been seen in female university modern dancers in the U.S.,[6,7] female university dancers in South Africa training in mixed-dance styles,[8] commercial jazz dancers† at a Los Angeles university,[9] as well as among female dancers in non-Western dance styles such as North Indian Kathak dance.[10]

Currently, research on male dancers is limited. Available information shows that males are not immune to developing disordered eating and eating disorders,[3,11] though they may be at lower risk than females. We have no data on eating disorder prevalence estimates or risk in dancers who do not fit the male/female binary, but there is growing evidence that transgender and gender nonbinary individuals are at higher risk for eating disorders than their cisgender peers.[12] We need more studies including dancers of all genders, with more racial and ethnic diversity represented and further data on genres besides ballet. Current research offers us a narrow view of eating disorders in dancers, which is also reflective of the lack of diversity in dance, especially in ballet. Having a greater understanding of how factors such as race, ethnicity, gender, sexual orientation, socioeconomic status, dance style, and other attributes influence eating disorder risk is critical to developing effective prevention programs.

Much of the available research on eating disorders in dancers is also quite dated. We don't have data to tell us if rates of eating disorders in dancers are changing. Research not specific to dancers shows that the prevalence of eating disorders more than doubled globally between 2000 and 2018.[13] There is no evidence to suggest that this isn't the case in the dance world as well. Of note, these results do not include disordered eating and were pre-COVID-19. Recent studies have found a worrying increase in eating disorders during the coronavirus pandemic.[14,15]

Despite research limitations, it's evident that eating disorders and disordered eating are much too common among dancers. We all have a role to play in changing this.

Factors That Increase Risk

Sarah is a 15-year-old contemporary dancer. She is a straight-A student and prides herself on always giving 150% to everything she does. All her friends are dancers, and her life revolves around dance—school, dance classes, rehearsal, homework, watch dance videos, stretch, sleep, repeat. Her best friend, Amy, recently got the "fat talk" at their dance studio. Their teacher told Amy that she needed to lose weight before audition season. Friends, family, and teachers have always told Sarah how lucky she is to be so skinny, but no one has said that to her in a while. Sarah can feel her body changing and fears her own "fat talk" is coming soon. When Amy starts counting calories and cutting out carbs, Sarah decides to do the same. They share their calorie goals to encourage each other, and Sarah makes sure she always eats less and does more exercise than her friend. As Sarah loses weight, she is told how great she looks, receives praise on how her dancing has improved, and gets cast as the lead in the upcoming performance. Even though Sarah finds herself thinking about food all the time and feels dizzy in class, she sees how her hard work to change her body is paying off and knows she can't stop.

"Genetics loads the gun but the environment pulls the trigger." This quote from Dr. Judith Stern[16] is a powerful and accurate analogy (though I'm not a fan of the violent imagery). Eating disorders are not a choice. Various predisposing and precipitating factors come together and contribute to their development. Dance culture and the dance environment, especially in certain genres like ballet, can create a perfect storm of risk.

Sarah's story illustrates some of the biological, psychological, and environmental risk factors common in dance. One of the difficulties in the prevention and early identification of eating disorders in dancers is that many of the traits and behaviors that make someone a good dancer are also characteristic of eating disorders.[17] Table 3.1 highlights some of these similarities. For example, like Sarah, dancers must be committed to their training and are often expected, or believe they are expected, to do "whatever it takes" to make it as a dancer. A dancer who trains harder than anyone else, relentlessly pursues perfection, does what they are told without questioning, and ignores pain is praised. Some of these qualities are necessary. Dance requires hard work, discipline, and sacrifice. Striving for perfection is how dancers hone their art, and every dancer must perform despite pain at times. However, there is a fine line between the necessary traits to succeed as a dancer and problematic behaviors that can harm physical and mental health. We need to help dancers understand this line: to know when they need to push themselves and when they need to respect their body's limits, to recognize the times that more is not better and may actually be harmful, to know when to trust what is being asked of them and when to use their voice to advocate for themselves.

Table 3.1 Similarities Between Dancer Traits and Eating Disorder Characteristics

Dancer Trait	Eating Disorder Trait
Commitment to training	Excessive/compulsive exercise
Mental toughness	Rigid self-denial/self-discipline
Pursuit of excellence	Perfectionism
Coachable	Overcompliance
Perform despite pain	Denial of discomfort

Adapted from Thompson and Sherman.[17]

Table 3.2 Factors That Increase Risk of Eating Disorders (EDs)

Risk Factor	Notes
Age	Although EDs can occur at any age, they frequently develop in the teen years to early twenties.
Gender	EDs affect all genders, but females are at somewhat higher risk than males, and transgender/gender non-binary individuals may be at higher risk than their cisgender peers.[12]
Family history	Having a close relative with an ED or another mental health condition (e.g., depression, anxiety, addiction) increases risk.
Mental health conditions	Having another mental health condition (e.g., depression, anxiety, obsessive compulsive disorder, post-traumatic stress disorder) increases risk.
Trauma	Experiences of trauma (e.g., emotional, physical, or sexual abuse, neglect, loss, bullying), particularly in childhood, are associated with EDs.[18,19]
Low self-esteem	Multiple studies have linked low self-esteem with ED risk.[20]

Adapted from Mehler and Andersen[21] and National Eating Disorders Association (NEDA)[22] with additional sources as indicated.

Table 3.2 describes general risk factors that increase the likelihood of eating disorders. Although most of these cannot be changed, it's useful to be aware of them to better understand how and why an eating disorder may develop and to inform and improve prevention and early intervention efforts. Table 3.3 lists risk factors for eating disorders common among dancers, which are all potentially modifiable. We can teach dancers about the harms of dieting and under-fueling and help them learn how to nourish their bodies properly. We can reduce dancers' exposure to harmful messages about food and bodies and replace them with messages and practices that help dancers develop more positive and resilient body image. And we can all work together to challenge the often-unrealistic standards of thinness that exist in the dance world.

Types of Eating Disorders

Below are brief descriptions of eating disorders that are common in dancers (adapted from the DSM-5 Guidebook[23] and Academy for Eating Disorders guides[24,25]). This information is provided to give a better understanding of the behaviors and beliefs that your dancers may be dealing with. It is not intended to be used to diagnose a dancer with an eating disorder, which is not your responsibility unless it is within the scope of your profession (e.g., you are a doctor, therapist, or eating disorder specialist).

Table 3.3 Eating Disorder (ED) Risk Factors Common in Dance

Risk Factor	Notes
Dieting	One of the most common and preventable precursors to developing an eating disorder.
Negative energy balance	May be intentional (e.g., from dieting) or unintentional (e.g., from illness or not eating enough for the dancer's activity level).
Personality traits	Traits such as perfectionism and rigid thinking are linked to EDs.[22] We may not be able to eliminate these traits, but we can help dancers learn how to recognize and manage them.
Body image dissatisfaction	Body image dissatisfaction is very common among dancers, may present differently depending on gender, and is influenced by the factors listed below.
Internalization of the thin ideal	When dancers accept the value that society and the dance world give to thinness and apply this value to themselves.
Exposure to harmful messages about food and body	This includes messages that reinforce the idea that thinner is better or ascribe moral value to food choices.
In an activity or profession that requires/favors a thin/lean body or low weight	Dancers, like other aesthetic athletes, are at increased risk for EDs based on weight and/or body size expectations in the field, though this varies somewhat by dance genre.
Being criticized about weight/body	Criticism or teasing about body size, shape, or weight by teachers, family, or friends increases the risk of EDs.
Peer pressure	Dancers may be influenced by friends and peers to diet or engage in other disordered eating or weight control behaviors.
Comparison	Engaging in body- and eating-related comparison to others is common among dancers—in the dance environment and especially on social media.

Anorexia Nervosa (AN) is characterized by restriction of energy (aka calorie) intake relative to needs which leads to a significantly low body weight—i.e., a weight lower than is expected based on the dancer's age, sex, developmental trajectory, and health. There are two subtypes of AN: restricting type (characterized by caloric restriction) and binge-eating/purging type (characterized by caloric restriction and recurrent episodes of binge eating or purging behaviors such as vomiting, laxative abuse, or diuretic abuse). Excessive exercise may occur in either subtype. AN is also associated with:

• Weight loss or lack of adequate weight gain and growth in children and adolescents

- Intense fear of gaining weight or becoming fat
- Persistent use of behaviors that interfere with achieving and maintaining a biologically appropriate weight
- Body image distortions (e.g., experiencing their body as larger than it is)
- Self-worth excessively influenced by body weight, size, and/or shape
- Not recognizing the seriousness of their behaviors and/or condition

Atypical Anorexia Nervosa (AAN) includes all the same behaviors and characteristics as AN, except the dancer's weight is within or above the "normal" range. Although the dancer may not appear "underweight," their weight may be too low compared to the weight at which their body functions best. Although AAN technically falls under the other specified feeding or eating disorder diagnosis described below, it is really just another presentation of AN. Atypical anorexia nervosa is just as serious as AN, carrying the same risks to physical and mental health, yet it is less likely to be identified and treated appropriately due to pervasive weight stigma in the medical and mental health fields[26] and in the dance world. The atypical label is also inaccurate because AAN is actually far more prevalent than AN,[26] and therefore not atypical at all.

Bulimia Nervosa (BN) is characterized by recurrent cycles of binge eating (i.e., eating a large quantity of food in a relatively short period of time) and compensatory behaviors such as self-induced vomiting, laxative abuse, diuretic abuse, fasting, or excessive exercise. BN is also associated with:

- Feeling out of control during binge episodes
- Intense fear of weight gain
- Compensatory behaviors motivated by a desire to counteract binges and prevent weight gain
- Self-worth excessively influenced by body weight, size, and/or shape
- Weight often within or above "normal" range

Binge Eating Disorder (BED) is characterized by recurrent episodes of binge eating without the use of compensatory behaviors. Many people overeat occasionally and may feel uncomfortably full as a result. "Over"-eating is relative but basically means eating more food than your body needs or feels comfortable consuming at a given time. Binge eating is different because it happens more habitually and involves significantly more psychological distress. Other characteristics of BED include:

- Feeling out of control during binge episodes
- Binges are associated with eating quickly, alone, in the absence of hunger, or until uncomfortably full
- Feelings of guilt, shame, embarrassment, disgust, or depression after a binge
- Self-worth excessively influenced by body weight, size, and/or shape (in many cases)[27]

- Restrictive eating is usually present and is a major contributing factor to binges
- Can be any weight or size

As mentioned above, many people with BED also restrict their intake in some way, are inadequately nourished, or have a deprivation or compensatory mindset with food. Addressing the restriction portion of the restrict/binge cycle is an essential part of recovery. Tragically, this aspect is not only frequently neglected, but recommendations to restrict food further are often given to individuals with BED, which causes further harm.

Other Specified Feeding or Eating Disorder (OSFED) is the diagnosis used when a dancer meets some, but not all, of the criteria for one of the other eating disorders. OSFED causes significant physical and psychological problems and distress and is no less serious than the other diagnoses. Examples of OSFED include:

- AAN
- BN of low frequency and/or limited duration
- BED of low frequency and/or limited duration

Other specified feeding or eating disorder was previously EDNOS before the diagnostic criteria for eating disorders changed in 2013. As mentioned previously, EDNOS (now OSFED) is likely the most common eating disorder in dancers. However, of note, BED would have been included under EDNOS in most of the existing studies on eating disorders in dancers, rather than as a separate diagnosis, as it is now.

Orthorexia is not currently recognized as an official eating disorder diagnosis but is worth mentioning here. The term "orthorexia nervosa" was first coined by Dr. Steven Bratman to describe eating behaviors that, although motivated by the desire to be healthy, become obsessive and harmful to the individual's health and well-being. Food rules and rigidity can impact all aspects of the individual's life and lead to malnutrition.[28] Behaviors associated with orthorexia vary from person to person, but often include (adapted from Dunn and Bratman[28] and NEDA[29]):

- Overconcern with ingredients and nutrients
- Spending a lot of time thinking about and evaluating food choices and/or in food preparation
- Elimination of foods that are not considered "healthy," "pure," or "clean"
- Experiencing significant distress when safe/allowed foods are not available
- Fear of disease and/or feelings of anxiety or guilt if self-imposed rules are not followed
- Weight loss and body image concerns may or may not be present

There are clear differences between the eating disorder types as described above, but many similarities exist as well. Especially in dancers, eating disorders usually involve overconcern with weight, body size, and/or shape. It's also common for dancers to have negative body image and a sense of self-worth excessively influenced by beliefs about their body. Denial of the severity of the situation is frequently present and influenced by an environment that tolerates and even encourages disordered habits. One of the most critical things to remember is that a dancer can have any of the eating disorders at any weight or size. They may be in a larger body and have anorexia nervosa or be in a smaller body and have BED. You cannot tell if a dancer has an eating disorder, or the severity of the eating disorder, based on their appearance.

Signs and Symptoms of Eating Disorders

If you work with dancers, you will encounter eating disorders. But how can you tell which dancers may be dealing with these serious conditions? Most people think of low weight or noticeable weight loss as red flags that a dancer may need help, and these are the most common reasons dancers are referred to me by their school or company. I am thankful these dancers are being encouraged to get help. Weight loss and low weight in a dancer are concerning and absolutely warrant further assessment. And yet, if these are the only criteria being used to identify dancers who may have an eating disorder, you are missing the majority of dancers with eating disorders.

Brianna is a 19-year-old ballet dancer who was recently promoted from apprentice to corps in her company on the condition that she lose weight prior to the start of her contract. She is told that she should lose weight in a "healthy" way and warned not to lose too much because the artistic director doesn't like dancers who are "too thin." She is not given any specific guidance or a referral to a dietitian. Brianna does some research online and begins to eliminate foods and stops eating snacks, but her weight doesn't change much. She cuts her intake further, and eventually starts to binge at night which makes her feel guilty and disgusted with herself. Brianna's periods have never been regular, but they stop completely. Her foot pain worsens, and she is diagnosed with a stress fracture. She needs to take at least six weeks off from dancing, so she returns home to stay with her parents. Her mom notices how little Brianna is eating and how anxious she is at family meals, and becomes concerned that her daughter may have an eating disorder. Brianna goes to see her primary care doctor for an evaluation who tells her that her weight is too high for her to have an eating disorder and that it is normal for dancers not to get their periods. When her vital signs are checked, her heart rate is low, but the doctor says this is normal for athletes and sends her home with a low-calorie meal plan to help her reach her weight-loss goals.

Although eating disorders can cause life-threatening psychological and physical complications, the warning signs are frequently overlooked, even by medical and mental health professionals. Physical signs and symptoms are often dismissed or attributed to another cause, especially when dancers are at or above a "normal" weight. Brianna's doctor displays how a lack of training and understanding about eating disorders coupled with weight stigma causes harm. Her doctor not only fails to give her an accurate diagnosis and referrals for necessary treatment but makes comments and recommendations that reinforce the eating disorder and impede recovery.

Even when a comprehensive medical assessment is done, the consequences of an eating disorder do not always show up in testing. A dancer with a severe eating disorder may have normal blood work and other test results (e.g., bone density test), but normal results should not be interpreted to mean that the dancer is fine. The human body is amazingly well designed for survival. When the body is under-nourished, it will sacrifice non-essential functions to keep you alive. For example, the body will break down bone to release calcium so that blood levels stay in the necessary range, and it will decrease reproductive hormone production to conserve energy to maintain vital organ functions. Medical markers may appear "normal" for a short period of time or for an extended duration depending on the dancer's genetics; however, this does not mean the dancer's body is functioning normally or optimally. It's also important to know that not every aspect of physical health can be tested.

Expanding our understanding of how eating disorders manifest physically, mentally, and behaviorally can help in identifying dancers who may be at risk. Some signs/symptoms such as an adolescent falling off their usual growth curve, amenorrhea, stress fractures, or evidence of purging are red flags that warrant immediate evaluation and intervention. Other slightly less serious signs/symptoms, like fatigue or bloating, are generally considered caution flags indicating the need for additional monitoring or investigation.

Common physical, behavioral, and psychological signs and symptoms of eating disorders are listed below. Your relationship with the dancer will affect which signs and symptoms you may be able to observe. Healthcare professionals such as doctors and physical therapists are in a good position to identify many of the physical signs. A teacher who sees an adolescent dancer in a leotard and tights every day may notice body changes before parents do. Family members, friends, and peers may become aware of changes in a dancer's eating habits and mood before these issues are seen by studio staff. If you are on tour with a dancer, you may have an opportunity to observe eating and exercise behaviors that may not be spotted by a teacher who only sees the dancer in class a few times per week. Regardless of the capacity in which you train, care for, or interact with dancers, you can play an important part in identifying dancers who may have an eating disorder by familiarizing yourself with the following signs and symptoms.

Physical Signs and Symptoms

Table 3.4 shows how eating disorders can impact just about every body part and system. Prevention and early intervention are key to preventing these serious and sometimes irreversible consequences.

Table 3.4 Physical Signs and Symptoms of Eating Disorders

Head/Brain: dizziness, fainting, brain fog, headaches, difficulty sleeping
Face: swollen cheeks/glands
Mouth: loss of tooth enamel, tooth sensitivity, cavities, tooth discoloration, sores at corners of the mouth
Throat: frequent sore throat, blood in vomit, heartburn
Chest/Heart: chest pain, heart palpitations, slow heart rate, low blood pressure, significant increase in heart rate with mild exertion
Abdomen/Stomach/Intestines: abdominal pain/discomfort, bloating, constipation, diarrhea, early satiety
Body: weight loss/gain/fluctuation, lack of weight gain/growth or change from usual growth chart percentiles in children and adolescents, fatigue, get cold easily
Hands/Feet: cuts/calluses on back of hand, brittle nails, cold and blue hands/feet, swollen hands/feet
Muscles, Bones, and Joints: muscle weakness, muscle wasting, repeated/slow-healing injuries, reduced bone density, fractures
Hair and Skin: lanugo (growth of fine hair on face and body), hair loss/thinning, dry skin, slow wound healing, yellowish skin, bruise easily
Hormones: absent/irregular periods, low libido, infertility

Adapted from Mehler and Andersen,[21] Gaudiani,[26] and NEDA.[30]

Behavioral Signs and Symptoms

- Dieting, skipping meals, fasting
- Rigid food rules
- Restricted/reduced food intake ("I'm not hungry," "I just ate")
- Refusal of certain foods or food groups ("I don't/can't eat that")
- Excuses to avoid meals and situations involving food
- Food rituals (e.g., cutting food into small pieces, eating foods in a specific order)
- Frequent body checking (e.g., spending excessive time in front of the mirror and/or checking weight/measurements)
- Hiding or hoarding food, secret eating
- Use of diet pills or weight-loss supplements
- Misuse of laxatives, diuretics, or medications
- Excessive caffeine or fluid consumption
- Excessive gum chewing
- Eating an excessive quantity of food in a short period of time (you might see lots of empty food wrappers/containers)
- Frequent bathroom trips after meals (you might see signs of vomiting)
- Dressing in layers of clothing (to hide body or to stay warm)
- Withdrawal from friends and usual activities
- Compulsive/excessive exercise (despite injury, illness, fatigue, weather)
- Excessive movement (e.g., restlessness, fidgeting)[31]

Psychological Signs and Symptoms

- Obsessive thoughts
- Moodiness/irritability
- Depression
- Suicidal thoughts[24]
- Anxiety
- Feeling shame and guilt (especially related to food, eating, exercise and/or body weight/size)
- Body image dissatisfaction, body dysmorphia
- Difficulty concentrating
- Poor memory
- Increased preoccupation with weight, body size/shape, food, calories, exercise
- Decreased ability to be spontaneous/flexible (e.g., with meals/exercise)

Eating disorders often serve as coping mechanisms which may develop or flare up in times of stress. Although eating disorder behaviors are used to manage distress, the eating disorder itself usually increases stress, anxiety, and overwhelm, in part because of the effects of malnutrition on the brain. If you are aware that a dancer is dealing with difficult life circumstances, it may be helpful to pay extra attention to the presence of any warning signs and symptoms of a possible eating disorder. Understanding that a dancer's eating disorder may be the only way they know how to deal with painful emotions or exert some sense of control when they feel overwhelmed will help you intervene in an empathetic way that helps support their recovery.

What to Do (and Not Do) If You Suspect an Eating Disorder

You've noticed some concerning signs in a dancer and worry they may have an eating disorder. What do you do now? Ideally your dance school, company, or clinic has an eating disorder policy in place to guide your next steps. If you are a dance teacher or staff member and no policy exists, it may be beneficial to advocate for one. If you are in a leadership position, I recommend assembling a team including medical professionals, eating disorder specialists, legal advisors, and key members of your organization to help you develop appropriate eating disorder guidelines that fit your needs and resources.

An eating disorder policy outlines who should be involved and how the situation will be handled if there are concerns about a dancer, which helps to ensure consistency, manage expectations, and reduce stress for everyone involved. Table 3.5 provides additional details on some of the information to include in an eating disorder policy. If you are a parent, there's no need for a set protocol, but having an idea of how you will approach your dancer, what to say, and goals for the conversation are equally important.

Table 3.5 What to Include in an Eating Disorder Policy

Considerations	Notes
Who concerns should be reported to	Select a person(s) in your organization with whom teachers, staff, parents, and dancers themselves can confidentially share concerns.
Warning signs and symptoms	List physical, behavioral, and psychological warning signs and symptoms and categorize by risk level (e.g., red/yellow light or flag system).
Indications for intervention	The primary goal is early identification and intervention. Outline how signs and symptoms will be tracked. For example, all concerns will be reported to a member of the healthcare team or administration who is responsible for initiating further action when needed. Specify which warning signs require immediate action (e.g., red light/flags) and how many lower-risk signs (e.g., yellow light/flags) need to be identified to trigger an intervention.
Who will speak to the dancer	Designate an individual(s) who will speak to the dancer when disordered eating or an eating disorder is suspected. Specify when parents/guardians will be involved (e.g., in cases involving minors).
What will be said	Outline the approach and language to be used and not used.
Referral lists	Include a list of eating disorder specialists (dietitians, physicians, therapists, psychiatrists) for referrals. Consider including a letter template to provide to the healthcare professional requesting confirmation that the dancer is cleared to continue dancing/training and if any modifications are needed.
Follow-up procedures	Specify next steps to take and in what time frame if the dancer agrees to an evaluation or if they refuse to comply with the recommendation.
Prevention measures	Provide tools and recommendations for screening (e.g., who will screen dancers and how often). Outline practices and/or language to be avoided (e.g., commenting on a dancer's weight). Provide resources for further education on eating disorders and disordered eating.

For parents, teachers, and staff, your role is not to diagnose or treat the eating disorder or disordered eating. The objective of expressing your concerns to the dancer is to have them evaluated by a qualified professional to determine a diagnosis and appropriate treatment plan. The dancer should be referred to a specific healthcare professional (i.e., dietitian, psychotherapist, physician, psychiatrist) who specializes in eating disorders and preferably also has expertise or at least experience in working with dancers.

The goal is for the dancer to receive help as soon as possible. Don't delay the process by waiting until they agree to an evaluation before you begin searching for providers to refer them to. Do some research to compile a list of trusted healthcare professionals prior to speaking with the dancer. Unfortunately, many medical and mental health professionals, including doctors, lack training in eating disorders and even fewer have experience with both eating disorders/disordered eating and dance. Sending your dancer to the right provider is of utmost importance because seeking care from untrained or under-qualified professionals will impede treatment and recovery. Thankfully, if you are unable to find suitable providers locally, telehealth can greatly expand your options. The Appendix provides additional recommendations to help find a treatment team for your dancers.

Communicating with Your Dancer

If you are concerned that one of your dancers has an eating disorder or disordered eating, you may also be worried that you will say or do the wrong thing or make the situation worse. Here are some recommendations to guide your conversation with the dancer:

Where/when: Speak to the dancer in a private, quiet setting without disruptions when your time is not limited. For parents/caregivers, avoid expressing your concerns during mealtimes (choose a more neutral time/place instead).

Who: To help the dancer feel more comfortable, it is usually beneficial if the person speaking with the dancer has a good relationship with them but is not a person in a position of significant power (e.g., artistic director of the company). If your organization has a health and wellness team, it may be helpful if a member of this team (e.g., dietitian, therapist, physical therapist) leads or participates in the discussion. Those involved in the conversation should have basic training on eating disorders/disordered eating and feel comfortable speaking with the dancer about this sensitive issue. Maintain confidentiality to the extent possible and tell the dancer who you will be communicating what information with and why. Concerns and updates about the dancer should only be shared on a "need to know" basis. Parents/guardians of minors need to be involved, and teachers and choreographers working directly with the dancer may also need to be informed, especially if training or participation needs to be adjusted.

How: Be direct, compassionate, and supportive. Express your care and concern using "I" statements and non-judgmental language. Be patient and allow the dancer to share their thoughts and feelings. Keep in mind that this will likely be a difficult conversation for them and that they may be experiencing shame. Provide referrals to a specialist for further evaluation, which can be a member of your organization's health team (if available) or an outside professional. Ask if the dancer would like help with scheduling their appointment. Dancers may be most open to seeing a dietitian as it might feel less threatening and have less associated stigma. If the dancer prefers to select their own provider(s), give them guidance on the type of assessment required and, if the dancer agrees, you can offer to speak with the provider about your concerns.

What to say: Starting the conversation by simply inquiring how the dancer is doing can be a good entry point. Tell the dancer what you value about them as a dancer and as a person and that there is nothing more important than their health and well-being. You can then share your concerns. Try to focus more generally on the dancer's energy, fueling, nutrition status, or health instead of discussing specific eating disorder behaviors, which might increase feelings of shame or make them defensive. In most cases, it's better not to discuss weight. Telling a dancer that you are concerned about their weight gain/higher weight will be more harmful than helpful. However, in some situations, a dancer might benefit from hearing that their weight is too low and weight gain is necessary.

Some dancers believe that needing help is a sign of weakness or failure or that they don't deserve it because things aren't "that bad." Remind the dancer that eating and body image issues are common among dancers and you are here to support them in getting the care they need before things become worse. Everyone deserves help and asking for it and accepting it takes courage.

The language used when communicating with the dancer is key. Here are some specific examples of what you might say:

> *We've noticed that you seem to have less energy in class than usual (or you seem to be having a hard time finishing x variation recently or you are having a difficult time focusing or you seem to be training so hard to the point of diminishing returns). We are concerned and wanted to check in: how are you feeling?*

> *I've noticed you haven't been eating lunch with the other dancers (or that you've had a few injuries recently). I'm worried you might not be giving your body the fuel it needs to dance and function best. What do you think?*

> *We care about you and want you to be the healthiest dancer and person you can be. We think it would be helpful to see a dietitian/therapist/ doctor for an evaluation. How would you feel about that?*

Sometimes it's also useful to know what not to do in these situations:

- Don't accuse the dancer of having an eating disorder or confront them about specific eating disorder behaviors.
- Don't criticize, blame, threaten, or punish the dancer.
- Don't demand that the dancer change or fix the problem, especially without giving them resources.
- Don't minimize how serious and challenging an eating disorder is (e.g., don't suggest that the dancer just needs to eat more).
- Don't offer nutrition or therapeutic advice.

- Don't undermine the recovery process (e.g., by saying you want the dancer to gain weight, but not too much).

Hopefully, when you speak with the dancer, they will understand the cause for concern and agree to have the recommended evaluation. Unfortunately, things don't always go this way. The dancer may deny having a problem. "I'm fine" is a common and expected response. This type of pushback is a further indicator that your concerns are likely justified because most healthy dancers wouldn't have strong opposition to a medical or nutritional assessment.

It may take more than one conversation with the dancer before they agree to be evaluated. Parents of minors can insist on a medical appointment whereas dance schools and companies cannot force a dancer to see a doctor or other healthcare provider. Depending on the degree of concern and risk, if a dancer continues to refuse an evaluation, the school/company can ask for written clearance from a physician before the dancer will be allowed to continue training and performing. You might say to the dancer, "We hope that you are right and that everything is fine, but we need you to get a letter from your doctor confirming that you are healthy enough to continue dancing." The doctor's letter should also specify if the dancer is cleared for full or modified activity.

Your support of the dancer needs to be ongoing and not limited to just these initial conversations. Lack of follow-up may unintentionally convey acceptance of the eating disorder or send the message that you think the dancer is doing better (even if they aren't). Although you may not be responsible for diagnosing or treating the dancer for their eating disorder, your support and understanding is an integral part of a dancer's recovery process.

Eating Disorder Treatment for Dancers

Full recovery from an eating disorder is possible with proper treatment, and there are several options available for dancers. The type of treatment and level of care recommended are based on multiple factors including the severity of the dancer's eating disorder/disordered eating; their motivation level; their medical, nutritional, and psychological status; insurance coverage; and their financial situation which may impact the ability to pay for costly treatment. The goal of treatment is to provide the dancer with the level of support needed to help them recover while causing the least disruption to their life.

A multidisciplinary approach is best with a treatment team that includes a dietitian, psychotherapist, and physician (generally a primary care or internal medicine doctor) at minimum. In some cases, a psychiatrist, other providers, or therapeutic groups may be included as well. It is beyond the scope of this book to discuss various treatment modalities, but family-focused treatment, or at the very least family involvement, is often beneficial and necessary for younger dancers (if feasible and appropriate for their family circumstances).

It's helpful for a dancer's family, friends, teachers, and employers to understand what treatment may involve. If a dancer is medically stable, outpatient care with individual team members will typically be recommended first. This is the lowest level of care where the dancer will meet with their individual therapist and dietitian once to twice a week each and have medical and psychiatric appointments less frequently. As the dancer progresses in recovery, sessions with the therapist and dietitian may decrease in frequency, though it is important not to reduce support prematurely. Outpatient care requires as little as one to two hours per week, so dancers are often able to continue with their usual class, rehearsal, and performance schedule if they have been cleared to do so.

When a dancer is unable to make sufficient progress in the outpatient setting, their team will recommend a higher level of care. Figure 3.2 shows the different levels of eating disorder treatment beginning at the first level, outpatient, and increasing in structure and support to the highest level of care, inpatient hospitalization. A dancer may be able to continue dancing while in an intensive outpatient program (IOP), though the amount of activity is usually reduced. Any treatment levels higher than IOP will require the dancer to significantly reduce their dancing or, more than likely, take a break from dancing.

Dancers may not want to increase the level of treatment, especially when it interferes with their normal activities. However, delaying additional support when it is indicated will also delay, and perhaps even prevent, full recovery. Imagine that you have an infection that requires treatment with a 14-day course of antibiotics. You decide to take half the prescribed dose for just seven days. There's a good chance that your infection will not be cured and may worsen. You need the right dose of treatment for the right length of time to heal.

Dancing can be a powerful motivator during the recovery process, but some dancers will need to decrease or stop to recover. As discussed in Chapter 2, busy dance schedules can make it difficult for dancers to fuel their bodies optimally. Eating enough to support a high activity level plus the needs of weight restoration is even more challenging and may not be possible. In addition, dancers may struggle to improve their eating and relationship with food while immersed in a dance environment that negatively influences their beliefs and behaviors about food and bodies. The treatment team may make a recommendation for removal from dance based on the severity of the dancer's eating disorder, their medical status (e.g., weight, vital signs, labs), and their ability to make progress while still dancing. This decision is never made lightly. If a dancer is required to stop dancing, allow them to choose whether they want to watch classes and rehearsals. For some dancers, staying involved in this way helps them feel connected to dance and their peers. Others may feel more upset, stressed, or isolated if they are made to observe while unable to participate physically.

Removal from dance is not a sign of failure or a punishment. It shows that the dancer's treatment team and school/company prioritize the dancer's health. Viewing the eating disorder as an injury (eating disorders are metabolic injuries) can help with understanding the need to stop dancing to support healing. The goal is to get the dancer back to doing what they love as soon as they are in a place to do so in a safe and healthy way.

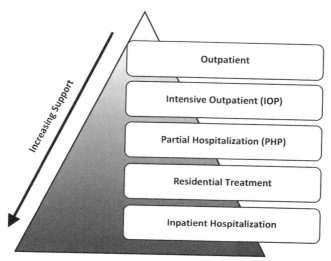

Outpatient: Once or twice weekly sessions with outpatient providers (e.g., dietitian, therapist).

Intensive Outpatient Program (IOP): Dancers participate in supported meals, individual therapeutic sessions, and groups for approximately 3 hours/day, 3-5 days/week.

Partial Hospitalization Program (PHP): aka Day Treatment. Dancers live at home or in housing near the treatment center and receive outpatient care 6-10 hours/day, 3-7 days/week.

Residential Treatment: Dancers live in and receive care in a non-hospital-based setting. Provides 24/7 supervision and medical monitoring as needed, but patients must be medically stable.

Inpatient Hospitalization: 24/7 clinical care provided in a hospital setting for patients who are medically or psychiatrically unstable.

Figure 3.2 Levels of Treatment for Eating Disorders.
Adapted from Anderson et al., 2017.[32]

As is the case with other injuries, a gradual return to dance is recommended with progression based on the dancer's ability to maintain treatment goals. Treatment contracts are sometimes helpful to outline specifically what is expected from the dancer to return to and continue dancing. Tools such as the Safe Exercise at Every Stage Athlete (SEES-A) Guideline, the Relative Energy Deficiency in Sport Clinical Assessment Tool (RED-S CAT™), and the Female and Male Athlete Triad Cumulative Risk Assessment tools and Clearance and Return-to-Play Guidelines can help guide decisions regarding removal from and return to dance (see the Appendix).

The Road to Recovery

The road to recovery from an eating disorder can be long and challenging. Making the decision to begin treatment is the first hurdle. Dancers may not think they have a problem or may not be ready to give up their eating disorder. Denial and ambivalence are expected and, contrary to popular belief, dancers don't need to feel fully ready to change in order to seek help. Having a trusted and experienced treatment team who understands the unique needs and pressures of being a dancer can help them find the motivation to take the first steps toward recovery.

Physical consequences of the eating disorder generally improve first (e.g., weight, vital signs), followed by behavioral aspects (e.g., restricting, compensatory behaviors), and then psychological recovery (e.g., changes in feelings and beliefs about food and body).[33] Full recovery can take several years, and there is an especially high risk of relapse in the first year after treatment.[34,35] If a dancer is underweight (i.e., at a weight lower than needed to support optimal physical and psychological health), gaining weight earlier in the treatment process and full weight restoration are important for recovery.[36] As mentioned in Chapter 2, it is the dancer's body (not their school/company, parents, or even medical providers) that determines the weight at which it functions best. However, it's critical that the dancer's treatment team not set estimated minimum weight targets too low as this will prevent full recovery and increase the chance of relapse.

Addressing body image dissatisfaction is a crucial, yet often neglected, part of recovery. Ongoing, long-term follow-up with treatment providers is also essential to prevent relapse. The healing process is not linear. Setbacks are inevitable, but if used as learning opportunities, they can help strengthen and further recovery. Intervening early when an eating disorder or disordered eating is suspected greatly improves the chances of recovery. Your support and understanding are also key. Check in with the dancer, ask how you can help, and be accepting of the body changes that may occur during the recovery process.

Communication between the treatment team and dance school/company can be helpful if the dancer (and parent/guardian in the case of minors) is open to it and provides written consent. This allows teachers and staff to cooperate with and reinforce treatment recommendations (e.g., modifications to training) and tell the treatment team about concerning behaviors or signs/symptoms they might not otherwise know about. Dancers need to be made aware of the reasons information will be shared and agree to what, when, and to whom it will be communicated. Decisions regarding information sharing should be guided by the dancer's wishes when possible and, to protect the therapeutic relationship, providers should only reveal pertinent details.

By preventing eating disorders and disordered eating from developing in the first place, we can spare dancers from having to go through a lengthy and arduous recovery process. Act II focuses on important aspects of prevention.

Main Pointes

- Dancers have a significantly higher risk of developing eating disorders than non-dancers.
- If you work with dancers, you will encounter eating disorders.
- Eating disorders can affect dancers of any genre or level.
- Although some key factors that contribute to eating disorders cannot be changed (e.g., genetics), many of the factors that increase the risk of dancers developing eating disorders are modifiable.
- You cannot tell whether a dancer has an eating disorder or the severity of an eating disorder based on their appearance.
- If weight loss and low weight are the only criteria being used to identify dancers who may have an eating disorder, you are missing most dancers with eating disorders.
- Everyone involved in the training and care of dancers has a key role to play in the early identification and intervention of eating disorders and disordered eating.
- It is not the role of dance educators, staff, and parents to diagnose or treat a dancer's eating disorder, but your support and understanding are an integral part of the recovery process.

Notes

When you imagine a dancer with an eating disorder, what comes to mind? How might these ideas help or hinder you in supporting a dancer who may have an eating disorder?

How have your own experiences in the dance world shaped your view of eating disorders?

If reading this chapter made you think that you might have disordered eating or an eating disorder, know that healing your relationship with food and your body is possible and it's never too late to get help.

Endnotes

* Based on now outdated diagnostic criteria, an eating disorder that didn't meet the full criteria for anorexia nervosa or bulimia nervosa was classified as EDNOS. This diagnosis does not mean the eating disorder was less severe.
† This study included female and male dancers (85 female, 4 male) but does not specify if any of the dancers who screened positive for an eating disorder were male.

References

1. Chesney E, Goodwin GM, Fazel S. Risks of all-cause and suicide mortality in mental disorders: A meta-review. *World Psychiatry*. 2014;13(2):153–160. doi:10.1002/wps.20128

2. Baker K. Heidi Guenther's short, tragic life – and death. April 4, 1999. Accessed November 27, 2022. https://www.sfgate.com/magazine/article/Heidi-Guenther-s-short-tragic-life-and-death-3490764.php
3. Arcelus J, Witcomb GL, Mitchell A. Prevalence of eating disorders amongst dancers: A systemic review and meta-analysis. *Eur Eat Disord Rev.* 2014;22(2):92–101. doi:10.1002/erv.2271
4. Ringham R, Klump K, Kaye W, et al. Eating disorder symptomatology among ballet dancers. *Int J Eat Disord.* 2006;39(6):503–508. doi:10.1002/eat.20299
5. Thomas JJ, Keel PK, Heatherton TF. Disordered eating attitudes and behaviors in ballet students: Examination of environmental and individual risk factors. *Int J Eat Disord.* 2005;38(3):263–268. doi:10.1002/eat.20185
6. Black DR, Larkin LJS, Coster DC, Leverenz LJ, Abood DA. Physiologic screening test for eating disorders/disordered eating among female collegiate athletes. *J Athl Train.* 2003;38(4):286–297.
7. Friesen KJ, Rozenek R, Clippinger K, Gunter K, Russo AC, Sklar SE. Bone mineral density and body composition of collegiate modern dancers. *J Dance Med Sci.* 2011;15(1):31–36.
8. Robbeson JG, Kruger HS, Wright HH. Disordered eating behavior, body image, and energy status of female student dancers. *Int J Sport Nutr Exerc Metab.* 2015;25(4):344–352. doi:10.1123/ijsnem.2013-0161
9. Heiland TL, Murray DS, Edley PP. Body image of dancers in Los Angeles: The cult of slenderness and media influence among dance students. *Res Dance Educ.* 2008;9(3):257–275. doi:10.1080/14647890802386932
10. Kulshreshtha M, Babu N, Goel NJ, Chandel S. Disordered eating attitudes and body shape concerns among North Indian Kathak dancers. *Int J Eat Disord.* 2021;54(2):148–154. doi:10.1002/eat.23425
11. Robson BE. Disordered eating in high school dance students: Some practical considerations. *J Dance Med Sci.* 2002;6(1):7–13.
12. Goetz TG, Wolk CB. Moving toward targeted eating disorder care for transgender, non-binary, and gender expansive patients in the United States. *Int J Eat Disord.* 2023;56(12):2210-2222. doi:10.1002/eat.24055
13. Galmiche M, Déchelotte P, Lambert G, Tavolacci MP. Prevalence of eating disorders over the 2000–2018 period: A systematic literature review. *Am J Clin Nutr.* 2019;109(5):1402–1413. doi:10.1093/ajcn/nqy342
14. Tavolacci MP, Ladner J, Déchelotte P. Sharp increase in eating disorders among university students since the COVID-19 pandemic. *Nutrients.* 2021;13(10):3415. doi:10.3390/nu13103415
15. Taquet M, Geddes JR, Luciano S, Harrison PJ. Incidence and outcomes of eating disorders during the COVID-19 pandemic. *Br J Psychiatry.* 2021;220(5):1–3. doi:10.1192/bjp.2021.105
16. Ramos RG, Olden K. Gene-environment interactions in the development of complex disease phenotypes. *Int J Environ Res Public Health.* 2008;5(1):4–11. doi:10.3390/ijerph5010004
17. Thompson RA, Sherman RT. "Good athlete" traits and characteristics of anorexia nervosa: Are they similar? *Eat Disord.* 1999;7(3):181–190. doi:10.1080/10640269908249284
18. Smyth JM, Heron KE, Wonderlich SA, Crosby RD, Thompson KM. The influence of reported trauma and adverse events on eating disturbance in young adults. *Int J Eat Disord.* 2008;41(3):195–202. doi:10.1002/eat.20490
19. Kjaersdam Telléus G, Lauritsen MB, Rodrigo-Domingo M. Prevalence of various traumatic events including sexual trauma in a clinical sample of patients with an eating disorder. *Front Psychol.* 2021;12:687452. doi:10.3389/fpsyg.2021.687452

20. Colmsee I-SO, Hank P, Bošnjak M. Low self-esteem as a risk factor for eating disorders. *Z Psychol*. 2021;229(1):48–69. doi:10.1027/2151-2604/a000433
21. Mehler PS, Andersen AE. *Eating Disorders: A Guide to Medical Care and Complications*. 2nd ed. Johns Hopkins University Press; 2010:288.
22. National Eating Disorders Association (NEDA). Risk factors. Accessed November 30, 2022. https://www.nationaleatingdisorders.org/risk-factors
23. Black DW, Grant JE. *DSM-5 Guidebook: The Essential Companion to the Diagnostic and Statistical Manual of Mental Disorders*. 1st ed. American Psychiatric Publishing; 2014:543.
24. Academy for Eating Disorders' (AED) Medical Care Standards Committee. Eating disorders: A guide to medical care. 4th ed. Published online 2021. Accessed December 1, 2022.
25. Academy for Eating Disorders Nutrition Working Group. Guidebook for nutrition treatment of eating disorders. Published online November 2020 Accessed December 1, 2022.
26. Gaudiani JL. *Sick Enough*. 1st ed. Routledge; 2018:276.
27. Hartmann AS, Lewer M, Vocks S. Body image disturbance and binge eating. In: Frank GKW, Berner LA, eds. *Binge Eating: A Transdiagnostic Psychopathology*. Springer International Publishing; 2020:181–192. doi:10.1007/978-3-030-43562-2_13
28. Dunn TM, Bratman S. On orthorexia nervosa: A review of the literature and proposed diagnostic criteria. *Eat Behav*. 2016;21:11–17. doi:10.1016/j.eatbeh.2015.12.006
29. National Eating Disorders Association (NEDA). Orthorexia. Accessed December 1, 2022. https://www.nationaleatingdisorders.org/learn/by-eating -disorder/other/orthorexia
30. National Eating Disorders Association (NEDA). Warning signs and symptoms. Accessed December 2, 2022. https://www.nationaleatingdisorders.org/warning -signs-and-symptoms
31. Casper RC. Restless activation and drive for activity in anorexia nervosa may reflect a disorder of energy homeostasis. *Int J Eat Disord*. 2016;49(8):750–752. doi:10.1002/eat.22575
32. Anderson LK, Reilly EE, Berner L, et al. Treating eating disorders at higher levels of care: Overview and challenges. *Curr Psychiatry Rep*. 2017;19(8):48. doi:10.1007/s11920-017-0796-4
33. Accurso EC, Sim L, Muhlheim L, Lebow J. Parents know best: Caregiver perspectives on eating disorder recovery. *Int J Eat Disord*. 2020;53(8):1252–1260. doi:10.1002/eat.23200
34. Strober M, Freeman R, Morrell W. The long-term course of severe anorexia nervosa in adolescents: Survival analysis of recovery, relapse, and outcome predictors over 10–15 years in a prospective study. *Int J Eat Disord*. 1997;22(4):339–360. doi:10.1002/(sici)1098-108x(199712)22:4<339::aid-eat1>3.0.co;2-n
35. Khalsa SS, Portnoff LC, McCurdy-McKinnon D, Feusner JD. What happens after treatment? A systematic review of relapse, remission, and recovery in anorexia nervosa. *J Eat Disord*. 2017;5:20. doi:10.1186/s40337-017-0145-3
36. Accurso EC, Ciao AC, Fitzsimmons-Craft EE, Lock JD, Le Grange D. Is weight gain really a catalyst for broader recovery?: The impact of weight gain on psychological symptoms in the treatment of adolescent anorexia nervosa. *Behav Res Ther*. 2014;56:1–6. doi:10.1016/j.brat.2014.02.006

Act II

Prevention, Prevention, Prevention

4 Prevention:
Why, Who, What, and When?

An ounce of prevention is worth a pound of cure.
~Benjamin Franklin

Why Focus on Prevention?

As you read in Act I, under-fueling,* disordered eating, and eating disorders can cause substantial harm to a dancer's health, well-being, and career. These issues can stunt dancers' physical, emotional, and artistic development and extinguish their love of dance. Eating disorders in particular are potentially life-threatening, and in most cases, life-pilfering—stealing a dancer's ability to be truly present and live life fully.

Recovery is possible with treatment and support, but the road to healing can be long, difficult, and financially burdensome. There may be several obstacles and delays to getting good care. Factors such as where a person lives, health insurance coverage, financial resources, and their support system impact treatment accessibility. A lack of training among medical providers in recognizing and assessing for eating disorders hinders early identification and intervention. Misinformation, stigma, and stereotypes† about eating disorders influence who is more likely to be diagnosed and referred for treatment.

Studies have shown that, despite a comparable prevalence of eating disorders[1] and similar or greater severity of symptoms, African American, Asian, and Latinx individuals are significantly less likely to be asked by their doctors about eating disorder symptoms, to be referred for further evaluation, or to get treatment than White individuals.[1,2] Nagata and colleagues found that the prevalence of disordered eating behaviors in young adults with higher weight was approximately double that of participants classified as "underweight" or "normal" weight, yet they were half as likely to receive an eating disorder diagnosis.[3] In addition, males with eating disorders are less likely to be diagnosed or receive treatment than females.[4] A lack of culturally sensitive and gender-inclusive and affirming treatment options are also barriers to getting appropriate care. Tragically, yet not surprisingly given the above factors, most people with eating disorders do not get the treatment they need.[4,5]

DOI: 10.4324/9781003366171-6

Although eating disorders are treatable illnesses, if they are not identified early and treatment is not utilized, they are more likely to become chronic, debilitating conditions with irreversible consequences. The goal of prevention is to spare dancers and their loved ones from this burden (while also acknowledging that we can make immense efforts to prevent eating disorders, and they can still emerge). Preventing under-fueling, eating disorders, and disordered eating is beneficial for schools and companies as these issues not only impact the health and well-being of your dancers, but can also affect their performance and your bottom line. Dancers with inadequate nutrition intake and/or disordered eating behaviors are more prone to injury[6-8] and injuries are a financial strain on dance companies.[9] When parents are choosing a dance school, most would prefer to send their child to a studio that nurtures, supports, and prioritizes dancer health than send their child to train in a place that has a reputation for being toxic. I've had several dancer clients (and/or their parents) make the decision to leave an unhealthy studio or company and move to one that was more conducive to helping the dancer stay physically and mentally healthy.

What We Know about Prevention

The good news is that prevention practices can simultaneously help dancers stay healthy and improve performance,[10] and we have evidence that prevention works. Studies have shown that prevention programs for dancers can improve their nutrition knowledge[11-14] and eating habits,[11] decrease disordered eating attitudes and behaviors,[15,16] as well as reduce risk factors for eating disorders such as body dissatisfaction,[13,16] drive for thinness,[13] and dieting/dietary restraint.[12,15,16]

Clinical psychologist and researcher Niva Piran implemented an effective eating disorder prevention program for 10–18-year-old male[‡] and female dancers in an elite ballet school.[15] This multifaceted program focused on changing the school environment by specifically addressing areas that teachers, staff, and students identified as having a negative influence on how dancers felt about their bodies. Piran worked with dancers and teachers/staff to make changes that helped create a more protective environment (e.g., dancers agreed not to engage in body-based teasing or comparison, teachers were prohibited from commenting on dancers' body shape). This decade-long prevention program significantly reduced disordered eating behaviors and unhealthy beliefs about eating and weight. In addition, there was a dramatic decrease in the prevalence of clinical eating disorders at the ballet school with virtually no new cases developing during the time of the program.[15] A follow-up study of Piran's prevention program found lasting benefits for participants 15 plus years later.[17]

Dance schools may acknowledge the need for a healthier dance environment yet remain hesitant to make changes for multiple reasons including a prevailing belief that they have a responsibility to prepare their dancers for the harsh reality of the dance world. Dance educators and leadership may think it's beneficial for dancers to "toughen up" in an environment that exposes them to the sometimes harmful expectations and practices they'll face in the "real world." However, Piran's results suggest the opposite. Older dancers in the program who were auditioning for company positions (i.e., facing considerable professional pressures) were able to maintain improvements in their eating behaviors and attitudes about their body.[15] According to Piran, this suggests that creating a healthier, more supportive subculture in a ballet school can benefit the dancers even when they leave that comparatively safer environment and enter a harsher dance world. In other words, we can give dancers education and support to counter harmful beliefs about food and bodies so that they don't become internalized and lead to the use of unhealthy behaviors in an effort to achieve the perceived ideal body.[15] We can protect dancers by providing them with a safe and nurturing space to train and develop.

An eating disorder prevention program for adolescent male and female elite athletes (including aesthetic sports like gymnastics) also showed encouraging results.[18] This one-year intervention was able to significantly reduce dieting and decrease the prevalence of eating disorders by 90% in female athletes. In addition, no new eating disorder cases developed in female or male athletes participating in the program (compared to eight new cases [13%] in females and one new case [<1%] in a male in the control groups). This prevention program included educational sessions for the athletes and coaches and also involved staff and parents.[18] Of note, both this program and Piran's were relatively long term, aimed at multiple targets (i.e., dancers/athletes and coaches/teachers/staff), and focused on systemic changes in the environment—an undoubtedly necessary aspect of successful prevention that makes individual changes possible and sustainable.

Who Should Participate in Prevention?

Alex is a 17-year-old modern dancer who has been exploring their gender identity and expression, which has made body image feel complicated. Teachers have never told them to lose weight directly, but Alex has noticed that thinner dancers are always selected for lead roles. Alex wants to lose weight to be more successful as a dancer and they decide to see a dietitian to do it the "right" way. The dietitian gives Alex a reduced-calorie meal plan and a list of foods to avoid and recommends tracking what they eat with a calorie counting app. Alex shares the plan with their mom to get help following it. Alex's mom tries to be supportive by getting rid of all the "junk food" in the house, pointing out foods that are just "empty calories," and frequently asking, "are you sure you want to eat that?" Alex tells their friends at the studio about their new diet plan and the dancers offer encouragement and tips to help. "You're being so good." "Try intermittent fasting—it helped my sister." "You're losing weight. You look great!" When

Alex goes to their doctor for their annual physical, the doctor notes that Alex dropped below their usual weight-for-age percentile on their growth chart, though Alex's weight is still above the 50th percentile. The doctor comments on Alex's weight loss. "I know dancers need to be skinny, and I'm not worried because your weight is still normal."

Alex's story shows the importance of everyone in a dancer's life participating in prevention. We cannot expect dancers to be physically and mentally healthy in an environment that accepts, ignores, or promotes harmful messages and practices around eating and weight. Living and training in an atmosphere that supports the development of healthy attitudes and behaviors is vital for preventing under-fueling, eating disorders, and disordered eating and is also critical to help dancers who are trying to recover from these conditions. Family, peers, teachers/staff, and healthcare providers can all play a role in helping or hindering dancers in building healthy habits and a positive relationship with food and their body.

Parents/Caregivers

A dancer's home environment exerts the earliest and usually most consistent influence on their eating habits and beliefs about food and bodies, giving parents/caregivers vital roles to play in prevention. Raising a healthy dancer amidst the powerful influences of diet culture and the pressures of the dance world is no easy feat. Parents/caregivers may wrestle with acknowledging the harms or futility of dieting yet not see any other options. You might believe that helping your child try to achieve the "ideal" body is the only way to spare them from hurtful body comments and criticisms. Like Alex's mom, you might think that if your child isn't happy with their body, you should help them change it.

Parents/caregivers may be dismayed to learn that encouraging or assisting a child in weight-loss attempts compromises their physical and mental health, even if it comes from a desire to help and protect. Adolescents who experience parental encouragement to diet are more likely to engage in unhealthy weight control behaviors and disordered eating (including binge eating), feel dissatisfied with their body, experience depression symptoms, and have lower self-esteem.[19] When these adolescents become adults, they have a higher risk of disordered eating, engaging in unhealthy weight control behaviors, and negative body image—in other words, the harmful impacts are enduring.[19] Of note, being encouraged to diet as an adolescent is also associated with higher weight as an adult.[19] It's important to consider the physiological and psychological effects of dieting and weight stigma (see Chapter 1) and also challenge the idea that being in a larger body is a "bad thing."

In addition, losing weight does not guarantee protection from hurtful body comments. As discussed in Chapter 5, any comments on body size/

shape, including those that praise thin bodies, can be detrimental. Supporting a child's desire to shrink their body sends the message that you agree that there is something wrong with them that needs to be fixed and perpetuates the harmful value system of diet and dance culture (i.e., a thinner body is better, healthier, more worthy).

A dancer's family can help prevent under-fueling, eating disorders, and disordered eating by countering (rather than reinforcing) diet culture messages and helping dancers connect with different values. Like in Piran's program[15] in which systemic changes in the dance school created a protective subculture, a healthy home environment can provide respite and insulate dancers from the negative influences they will encounter in society and in dance.[20] Ideally, dancers are able to grow up in a household where eating is nourishing and enjoyable (vs. a reward or punishment), foods are viewed as neutral (vs. categorized as good or bad), body diversity is appreciated (vs. idolizing thinness), bodies are valued for what they do (vs. what they look like), and dancers are taught to listen to, trust, and care for their body (vs. ignoring and constantly trying to change and manage it).

Healthcare Professionals

Healthcare spaces can also be safe and protective or (paradoxically) undermine dancers' health. Doctor appointments can feel like a minefield for someone trying to develop a healthy relationship with food and their body. Consider just some of the "mines" a dancer might face during a medical visit: a weight check and accompanying comments, the BMI poster on the wall, "healthy" eating and exercise advice (that can be quite disordered), and diet culture-laden small talk.

Even experienced doctors are often not well-versed in current research on the dangers of dieting or the harms of diet culture and the weight-centric approach.[21] Though physicians are in an optimal position to educate patients and their family about healthy habits and to identify risk factors and early signs and symptoms of under-fueling and eating disorders/disordered eating, unfortunately many lack adequate training in nutrition and eating disorders. Because of this gap in understanding and knowledge, even well-meaning physicians and other medical professionals often make harmful comments about weight, bodies, and nutrition. They may unintentionally reinforce disordered eating, miss warning signs and symptoms, dismiss concerns, and conclude that everything is "fine" when it isn't—losing key opportunities to assist in prevention.

Dance Educators/Staff and Peers

The dance school/company environment is one of the most critical areas to address in prevention.[17] Dancers often spend more time in the studio than they do at home, especially at advanced levels and even more so for dancers training away from home. Consequently, teachers, peers, and the school/company culture play a major role in shaping dancers' self-evaluation, body image, and behaviors—either positively or negatively.

It is well established that dancers are at high risk for under-fueling, eating disorders, and disordered eating (see Act I). Studies show that it is not dance training itself that is a risk factor for these issues, but rather, specific, and more importantly, modifiable characteristics of the dance setting.[22,23] A dance environment that exposes dancers to messages and practices that reinforce the thin ideal (e.g., body/weight-related comments/criticisms from teachers, weigh-ins, favoring thinner dancers) contributes to drive for thinness, body dissatisfaction, and eating disorders in dancers.[23]

As role models, mentors, and authority figures who dancers look up to and want to please, teachers exert powerful influence on how dancers feel about themselves as well as their behaviors.[20,24] Experiencing pressure from teachers about weight, appearance, or food choices is linked to a higher risk of eating disorders in dancers.[22] Dancers frequently identify teachers as a key factor contributing to their body dissatisfaction,[25] and some dancers report that teachers have a far greater impact on their body image than their parents do.[20]

Dancers' peers also carry significant influence. Negative body talk and comparison are common among dancers and contribute to body dissatisfaction.[20,26] In a study of female adolescent and young adult dancers, figure skaters, and runners, peers were the most frequently reported source of encouragement to lose weight/be thinner (followed by coaches, then parents).[27] Dancers often learn about dieting and disordered eating from their peers.[23] The acceptance, normalization, and even encouragement of these behaviors can contribute to a "contagion" effect[28] where diets and unhealthy weight control behaviors easily spread in a dance studio/school/company.

On the other hand, peers and teachers can serve as positive forces in prevention. A supportive teaching style that prioritizes dancers' health and well-being (rather than primarily emphasizing performance or focusing on body weight/size/shape) is protective.[24,29] Teachers can help dancers recognize and appreciate their own unique qualities, which in turn lessens harmful comparison.[30] Working with dancers in a way that enhances self-esteem, teaches dancers to believe in themselves,[30] and supports them in becoming the best dancer and person they can be is also beneficial.[10] In terms of peers, dancers remark that their supportive friendships with other dancers help them resist and recover from disordered eating behaviors.[20] In addition, school practices that encourage optimal fueling (e.g., scheduling adequate time for meal breaks, encouraging dancers to fuel and hydrate) are also protective.

Shifting Dance Culture

Including teachers, staff, and peers in prevention efforts is essential. Catching potential issues early is a key part of prevention and everyone in the dance environment can assist in early recognition and intervention for under-fueling, eating disorders, and disordered eating. Dancers with body image and eating concerns may confide in friends before they tell a parent, guardian, or teacher. Dancers may be the first to notice potentially problematic behaviors in their peers. Dancers need to know what to do and say in these situations. Peer involvement is also an essential part of maintaining positive changes that a prevention program brings about.[15] Although specific elements of prevention that dancers in a school/company receive will vary based on age and level, all dancers should be included rather than just a select group considered at highest risk. Involving everyone helps decrease shame and stigma, shows that leadership believes in the importance of this curriculum, and sends the message that all dancers have a valuable part to play in making their shared dance environment healthier and safer.

It's important to note that dancers recognize the difficulty (and perhaps futility) in trying to improve their eating habits and body image without support from those who train and employ them.[16] In feedback provided following an eating disorder prevention program conducted by Gorrell and colleagues (in which only professional dancers received the intervention), dancers requested that artistic and other staff be included in future iterations of the program in hopes that this might lead to more meaningful and sustainable systemic change.[16] As seen in the studies reviewed earlier in this chapter,[15,18] prevention programs targeting dancers/athletes plus teachers/coaches/staff had encouraging results. Their success may be in part due to an additive effect. Teachers/staff get the knowledge and skills they need to help dancers stay mentally and physically healthy, and dancers see that their teachers/staff support what they are learning and the changes they are being encouraged to make for their health and well-being.[31]

Although dancers acknowledge the need for systemic change in dance, they remain skeptical that such change will materialize, which can affect their motivation to make personal changes.[16] Why bother trying to eat better or feel better about their body in an atmosphere that will continue to reinforce the opposite? Dancers' skepticism is understandable. True prevention of under-fueling, eating disorders, and disordered eating in dancers will require change not just in individual schools and companies, but in the dance world as a whole.[15,20] Meaningful change will require a shifting of values across all stakeholders—a move away from an ultra-thin ideal prized at any cost and toward prioritizing dancers' physical and mental health. This type of change is possible but will undoubtedly be slow and face numerous hurdles. While we each do our part in fostering broader change, we must not lose sight of the importance of protecting and improving the health of dancers on a more micro level as well.[24]

What Should Prevention Include?

Prevention efforts should target multiple risk factors that contribute to under-fueling, eating disorders, and disordered eating. Risk factors for eating disorders fall into three categories:[§] predisposing factors (e.g., genetics, body dissatisfaction, perfectionism), precipitating or trigger factors (e.g., dieting, negative body comments, injury), and perpetuating or maintaining factors (e.g., teacher/parent approval, consequences of inadequate nutrition).[32] Predisposing factors increase the chances that a dancer will develop an eating disorder—these are the bullets that load the gun (to revisit the analogy from Chapter 3). The eating disorder begins when a precipitating factor(s) "pulls the trigger." Perpetuating factors support the continuance of the eating disorder, reinforcing unhealthy beliefs and behaviors.

Disordered eating and under-fueling share many of the same risk factors as eating disorders (eating disorders and disordered eating are also common causes of under-fueling). Some risk factors like genetics cannot be changed. However, many risk factors are modifiable, and focusing on these areas in prevention programs is useful (see Table 4.1). Perpetuating factors in the dance world, such as positive reinforcement of weight loss and endorsement of dieting behaviors, are especially important to address. If ignored, these factors can contribute to eating disorders, disordered eating, and under-fueling becoming chronic, making full recovery harder and less likely.

Dancers face different pressures and risk factors depending on their dance setting, so prevention efforts should be tailored to the issues most relevant to your dancers. Piran's prevention program[15] was guided by feedback from teachers, staff, and dancers. This collaborative approach enabled the program to address the specific needs of the dancers and the school and was a key part of its success.[15]

Prevention is more likely to be successful if dancers believe that their health is a priority for their school/company/family vs. an atmosphere where they feel their body size/shape and performance are valued above all else. Dancers also need to be encouraged to use their voice. They need an environment where they feel safe sharing their experiences and difficulties. They need to know that their concerns will be taken seriously.

Table 4.1 Modifiable Risk Factors to Target in Prevention

Predisposing Factors	*Trigger Factors*	*Maintaining Factors*
Body dissatisfaction Low self-esteem Perfectionism Peer pressure Media influence	Dieting Negative energy balance Comments/criticism about weight, body, eating Injury	Teacher/parent approval Failure to identify signs/symptoms Physical and psychological effects of under-fueling Lack of healthy coping skills

Adapted from Bratland-Sanda and Sundgot-Borgen.[32]

There are two main goals of prevention. Primary prevention efforts are aimed to prevent the development of disordered eating, eating disorders, and under-fueling.[33] Secondary prevention focuses on identifying early signs and symptoms of these conditions to allow for prompt intervention and prevent progression to more serious stages.[33] Education and screening are essential components of primary and secondary prevention, respectively.[34]

Education

There are three broad inter-related areas—restrictive eating practices/inadequate fueling, negative attitudes about weight/shape, and psychological risk factors—that should be addressed in educational programs, along with the factors that contribute to and exacerbate them. As illustrated in Figure 4.1, the goal of education is to provide dancers and those who train and care for them with the knowledge and tools they need to shift the balance away from eating disorders, disordered eating, and under-fueling toward healthy habits and a healthy mindset.

Education: Dancers

Increasing dancers' nutrition knowledge can help improve their eating habits and decrease disordered eating behaviors.[11,12,35]

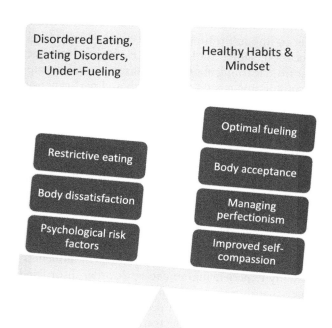

Figure 4.1 Shifting the Balance Toward Health.

Nutrition education for dancers should focus on helping them learn how to eat in a way that is nourishing, enjoyable, and supports their physical and mental health and performance. Dancers need education on topics such as what optimal fueling for dancers looks like, meal and snack planning for busy dance schedules, the harms of dieting and under-fueling, and how to sort nutrition fact from fiction.

Dancers' body image and their relationship with food impact how they nourish and care for themselves, which are important, yet often neglected, aspects to cover in educational sessions. Addressing body dissatisfaction and internalization of the thin ideal is essential. Dancers need guidance on how to develop a healthy and peaceful relationship with food and their body, reduce exposure to and counter harmful messages they encounter, build resiliency to negative body image, and do their part to create and maintain a supportive and protective dance environment.

Some may worry that talking to dancers about eating disorders causes eating disorders, yet eating disorders thrive in silence and isolation. Not discussing them sends the message that eating disorders are a taboo topic, which increases shame and stigma, hinders prevention, and creates barriers to early intervention. Instead, empowering dancers with knowledge can be an important component of prevention if careful attention is given to ensure that content is age appropriate, and that information is presented in a helpful rather than harmful way.

Currently there is no consensus on the best age to talk about eating disorders with dancers. However, given that adolescence is a peak period for eating disorder development, this is an important time for dancers to receive developmentally appropriate education. Older adolescents (i.e., high school age) and adult dancers can benefit from learning about eating disorder signs, symptoms, and consequences, including impacts on their health and performance, as long as this information is thoughtfully presented.[18,36-38] Behavioral aspects of eating disorders should be discussed with caution—providing essential information, not a how-to guide.[39] The use of images must be carefully considered (e.g., don't show pictures of emaciated individuals), and eating disorders should not be glamorized (e.g., by mentioning celebrities).[40] Stereotypes should be debunked by emphasizing that eating disorders affect all genders, ethnicities, and body sizes.[40,41] Dancers need to know that a variety of bio-psycho-social factors contribute to the development of eating disorders.[40,41] These conditions are not a choice, but they are preventable and treatable.

Reminding dancers that eating and body image concerns are common in the dance world can help to reduce shame, stigma, and feelings of aloneness. Even if a dancer isn't personally experiencing an eating disorder/disordered eating, there is a good chance that during their training and career they will encounter at least one peer who is, given the high prevalence of these issues in dancers. In addition, if dancers go on to become teachers, choreographers, leaders, or pursue another career working with dancers, knowledge about eating disorders is vital. Dancers need to know how to recognize eating disorders and disordered eating and what to do if they are concerned about themselves or someone they know. For those who may already be exhibiting disordered beliefs or behaviors, educational sessions can encourage them to seek help.

Younger adolescents benefit from learning about many of the same topics as older dancers,[42] but information needs to be suitable for a different level of understanding and maturity. Generally, for dancers under 12, education aimed at eating disorder prevention should focus on increasing protective factors (e.g., body appreciation, self-compassion) without explicitly discussing eating disorder symptoms or behaviors.[36] It's helpful for dancers of all ages to know that we are meant to feel peaceful and positive about food and our body and if that's not the case, it's good to talk to someone about it.[41]

Because eating disorders and disordered eating often serve as coping mechanisms, dancers need to learn healthier skills to manage difficult emotions and deal with life stressors like injury (see Chapters 7 and 9). Other valuable mental health topics for dancers include managing perfectionism, building self-compassion, how anxiety/depression can impact health and performance, and when seeking help is indicated. Additional suggested topics for educational sessions for dancers are listed in Table 4.2.

We need to normalize and encourage seeking help for eating, body image, and mental health issues sooner rather than later.

Table 4.2 Topics for Dancer Education

Optimal fueling for dancers
Meal timing to enhance performance and recovery
Meal planning (including how to put together nourishing meals and snacks for busy dance schedules)
Dietary supplements
Debunking nutrition myths
How to develop a healthy relationship with food, body, and exercise
Harms of dieting for performance and health
Signs, symptoms, and consequences of under-fueling (including education on Female Athlete Triad, Male Athlete Triad, RED-S)
Signs, symptoms, and consequences of eating disorders
How to get help for under-fueling, eating disorders, and disordered eating
Body appreciation and body acceptance
Life skills (e.g., grocery shopping, cooking basics, budgeting)
Media literacy
Injury prevention and recovery
Self-care (including sleep, stress management, and healthy coping tools)
Other mental health topics: self-esteem, self-compassion, anxiety/depression, perfectionism, managing performance/audition/career-related anxiety

It is courageous, not shameful, to get support, and dancers don't need to wait until they feel things are "bad enough." Educational sessions for dancers are usually given in a group setting, which provides social support[43] and can enhance learning (e.g., through group discussion)[44] but does not allow the individual concerns of dancers to be adequately assessed or addressed. The fewer barriers to dancers getting additional help the better. A list of resources (e.g., contact information for recommended providers) should be provided in educational sessions[40] and be available in other easily accessible areas such as in student handbooks or dressing rooms. It's also helpful if dancers are offered the opportunity to meet with a dietitian and therapist one-on-one. If a school/company has a dietitian and/or therapist on staff, it's preferable for dancers to be able to communicate with these providers directly vs. having to go through a teacher or other artistic staff/leadership. Ideally, all dancers are given the option for individual nutrition and therapy sessions to help reduce stigma and increase the chances that those who need help will be able to access it. If this is cost prohibitive, finding ways to reduce financial obstacles to getting help is important, perhaps by providing a limited number of sessions at low or no cost to dancers at higher risk.

Education: Teachers and Staff

As mentioned earlier, prevention programs will be more effective if dancers trust that teachers and staff support the education dancers are receiving. However, in some dance settings, having teachers or artistic staff present during sessions may limit dancers' openness and comfort in sharing or asking questions. It may be better to have teachers/staff introduce sessions, explain the value of what dancers are learning, and let dancers know that teachers/staff will receive education to complement the work the dancers are doing.

Teachers and staff benefit from much of the same education that dancers receive (see Table 4.2) with topics tailored to their role (e.g., how to communicate with dancers in a way that doesn't reinforce negative body image or contribute to disordered eating). Education on risk factors, signs, and symptoms of eating disorders/disordered eating and guidance on what to do and what not to do when concerned about a dancer should be mandatory for all teachers and support staff.[45] Sessions on these topics should be repeated regularly to reinforce concepts,[45] promote ongoing discussions about school/company-specific issues that need to be addressed, and reach new teachers/staff. All staff members can benefit from educational sessions, but it's especially important to include those who have interactions with dancers that provide opportunities to participate directly in prevention and early recognition (e.g., residence hall staff, costume shop employees, catering team, Pilates and conditioning teachers, physical therapists, etc.).

Education: Parents/Caregivers

Including parents in prevention efforts is helpful as well. Inform parents about what dancers are learning so they can reinforce protective messaging and practices, and if possible, provide parents with their own educational sessions. Parents need to know how to identify signs and symptoms of under-fueling and eating disorders/disordered eating and how to get help for and support their child if they are dealing with these issues. Other important topics for parents include nutrition needs of growing and developing dancers, nourishing meal and snack ideas, how to insulate dancers from harmful diet culture messages, and how to help dancers build self-compassion and develop healthy coping skills.

Education: Healthcare Professionals

Any healthcare professional (physician, dietitian, psychotherapist, physical therapist, athletic trainer, etc.) working with dancers needs at least basic education on eating disorders[45] to decrease the chances of inadvertently causing harm. Unfortunately, too few providers receive this necessary training.[46] Studios/companies with on-site or affiliated healthcare professionals should include them in staff educational sessions. Providers who do not receive this training where they work need to seek out their own continuing education and/or consultation/supervision in the recognition and management of eating disorders, disordered eating, and under-fueling.[45] Even those of us who specialize in these areas need to continue our learning and professional development to stay updated with new research and best practices to help dancers.

Teachers/staff, parents, and healthcare professionals all need to know how to help reduce rather than exacerbate risk factors such as body dissatisfaction, weight pressures, thin-ideal internalization, harmful dieting practices, and low self-esteem. Evaluating weight biases and exploring how personal experiences with food and body might impact our work with dancers is important for anyone involved in their training and care. Additional guidance to help create a protective environment is provided in Chapter 5.

Additional Recommendations for Educational Programs

Studies on successful prevention programs[15,16,18,31,47] offer valuable insights on ways to make prevention efforts more effective. Based on this research, as well as feedback received from workshops I've delivered to dancers, teachers/staff, parents, and healthcare professionals, here are some additional recommendations to help guide you. Educational programs for dancers should be:

- Mandatory
- Interactive

- Incorporated into training curriculum or on paid time for professionals
- Tailored to the unique needs of dancers
- Ongoing and include multiple sessions

Requiring all dancers to attend educational activities helps reduce stigma and social barriers to change. Incorporating sessions into training or paid time sends the message that taking care of one's physical and mental health is an integral part of being a dancer. Multiple sessions are needed because all pertinent subjects cannot be effectively covered in a single seminar. One-off sessions are also unlikely to lead to significant or sustainable changes in knowledge, attitudes, or behaviors.[47] Dancers need repetition and reinforcement of topics, especially to promote change in how they care for themselves and feel about food and their body. In addition, the more these subjects are repeated, the more likely they are to feel neutral instead of highly charged. The benefits of prevention programs typically decrease over time after the intervention ends.[11,14,18] Therefore, ongoing efforts are needed to maintain improvements.

Group sessions should be divided by age so that topics can be presented in a developmentally appropriate way and to help dancers feel more comfortable participating. Group size is an important consideration as well. Large and small groups each have advantages and disadvantages. Some dancers may feel more at ease in larger groups where there is less pressure to participate.[48] Larger group sessions are also more cost-effective. Alternatively, in my experience, smaller groups (8–20 participants) facilitate discussion and allow for more interactive activities which enhance learning.[47]

It is beneficial to consider gender when offering sessions. For example, exploring ways that dancers can collaborate to create a protective environment (e.g., no negative body talk or diet talk, no body or weight-based teasing) is helpful to do in mixed groups.[49] On the other hand, dancers (especially adolescents) might be more open to discussing sensitive topics like body image, pubertal body changes, or menstruation in gender-specific groups.[40,49] Although more research is needed to better understand risk factors for eating disorders, disordered eating, and under-fueling in males and other genders, including some sessions with gender-specific areas of focus may be useful (e.g., pressure to attain an ultra-thin physique for female dancers, pressure to achieve "ideal" musculature in male dancers,[49] unique body image pressures in non-binary dancers).

Selecting Education Providers

You find out that your dancer will attend a nutrition seminar during their summer intensive—that's a good thing, right? It depends on who is giving the session, what is being taught, and how. I've had many dancer clients share what they've been told in nutrition presentations given at their dance studios: Dancers shouldn't eat dairy or gluten because these foods cause inflammation. Dancers should eat only whole foods, nothing processed. Dancers shouldn't drink their calories. These recommendations are problematic for many reasons. They are inaccurate. They promote a one-size-fits-all approach that doesn't account for varying needs, preferences, or resources. And most importantly, giving dancers (a population at high risk for eating disorders, disordered eating, and under-fueling) this type of restrictive diet advice is harmful, especially in a group setting.

Education can be a key part of prevention, but only if the content is appropriate and presented in a way that is not detrimental. Choosing who will provide education to your dancers is critical. Presenters need to be good role models with eating and body image, so they don't disseminate their weight bias or harmful beliefs about food.[39,41] If the person leading the educational session has outside interactions with the dancers, consistency in messaging is important. For example, if a teacher or health coach speaks about body acceptance and students have heard them making negative body comments, the presenter will seem untrustworthy and their message inauthentic.[41]

Educational sessions should be led by qualified health professionals rather than a teacher or other staff member without adequate training in the areas that will be discussed.[14,47] Sessions on optimal fueling for dancers and other nutrition-related topics should be given by a Registered Dietitian (aka Registered Dietitian Nutritionist).** In the U.S., the title "nutritionist" is not regulated and does not guarantee any specific training or qualifications (i.e., anyone can call themselves a nutritionist).[50] In addition, educational requirements to become certified as a health or nutrition coach are far less rigorous and extensive than those needed to become a Registered Dietitian. Mental health topics such as self-esteem, perfectionism, stress management, depression, and anxiety are best covered by a qualified mental health professional (e.g., psychologist, social worker, marriage and family therapist, licensed mental health counselor, etc.).[51] Sessions on body image and eating disorders/disordered eating can be led by either Registered Dietitians or mental health professionals (preferably both for greater effect),[43] and presenters should have expertise in these areas.

Unfortunately, checking qualifications is not enough to ensure that you have found the best professional to teach your dancers about these sensitive topics. Asking many of the same questions about experience, training, philosophy, and approach listed in the Guidance for Finding Treatment Providers section of the Appendix will help you select an education provider. Inquire about what material will be presented to dancers and how (Chapter 5 provides recommendations on language and approach). Dancers will be most receptive to information that addresses their unique needs and challenges. So preferably, educational providers have experience working with dancers. In addition, providers who specialize in eating disorders as well as a weight-inclusive, non-diet approach are more likely to present material in a way that is protective for this vulnerable population.

Screening

Early recognition and prompt intervention for disordered eating, eating disorders, and under-fueling are key components of preventing these conditions from progressing in severity and chronicity. Unfortunately, dancers with eating disorders/disordered eating and those who are under-fueling rarely self-identify.[34] Dancers may not realize there is a problem. They may not believe it is serious enough to ask for help or understand the impacts on their health and performance. They may be embarrassed, ashamed, or afraid to let anyone know because they fear what addressing these issues may entail (e.g., weight gain, being removed from dance, losing something that helps them cope with difficult feelings). The normalization of dieting and disordered eating behaviors in diet culture and in dance as well as the similarities between eating disorder characteristics and dancer traits (see Chapter 3) also hinder early identification. For these reasons, specifically screening dancers for disordered eating, eating disorders, and inadequate nutrition is beneficial.[34]

Guidelines for screening for under-fueling (as well as signs and symptoms of the Triad and RED-S) were discussed in Chapter 2. There are several short, easy-to-use tools that can be used to screen[††] for eating disorder risk such as the Eating Disorder Examination Questionnaire Short (EDE-QS),[52] Eating Disorders Screen for Athletes (EDSA),[53] and the Eating disorder Screen for Primary care (ESP).[54] Screening questionnaires can be given to dancers to complete prior to healthcare visits (e.g., included as part of intake forms), which saves time for providers and may help dancers feel more comfortable disclosing disordered thoughts and behaviors than if they are asked about them face-to-face.[34,55] Providers can score the screen before meeting with the dancer, and if the screen is positive (i.e., indicates a possible eating disorder), next steps for further evaluation and management can be discussed.

There are also brief online screening tools like the InsideOut Institute Screener[56] that dancers can be encouraged to complete. The downside to an anonymous online tool is that if a dancer screens positive, providers can only give follow-up recommendations if the dancer shares the results. Though beyond the scope of this book to cover in detail, screening dancers for other mental health concerns (e.g., anxiety, depression, chronic stress) is also important,[57] as psychological issues can contribute to under-fueling and eating disorders/disordered eating[6,45] and also independently impact dancers' health. The Appendix provides links to the screening tools mentioned here.

Medical and mental health appointments provide excellent opportunities to incorporate regular screenings. Although it's not necessary to be a health professional to administer a screen (e.g., EDSA was developed for coaches to use[58]), it may be preferable considering the nature of the information collected and its purpose. No matter who is conducting the screening or asking the dancer to complete a self-screen, there needs to be a plan in place for what to do next[10] (i.e., who will review and score the screen, determine if follow-up is needed, communicate findings with the dancer, etc.). In most cases, a dancer who screens positive should be referred to an experienced specialist (dietitian, therapist, physician) who will do a more thorough assessment and determine a treatment plan, unless the person doing the screening is also qualified to conduct these next steps. Dancers should be given a list of potential specialists to see, either members of your school/company's health team or outside providers. The purpose of screening is early identification and intervention, so it's important to check back in with the dancer to make sure they follow through with recommendations sooner rather than later.

If your school/company has a dietitian and therapist on staff, offering dancers brief individual nutrition and mental health screening sessions, perhaps at the start of each semester or season, can be beneficial. Individual screening visits are a good way to identify potential issues and begin building a relationship with providers so dancers feel more comfortable reaching out to them if future issues arise. Although there are existing tools to screen for low energy availability,[59,60] a more in-depth nutrition assessment by a dietitian is the best way to evaluate the adequacy of a dancer's intake. One-on-one sessions also allow for a more nuanced and gentle approach which may feel less threatening and increase the likelihood of dancers sharing concerns.[34] Providers who specialize in eating disorders and working with dancers are skilled at picking up on subtext, identifying early indicators of problematic beliefs and behaviors, and asking questions in a way that makes dancers feel validated and safe enough to be open.

Dancers should always be made aware of the purpose of screenings (e.g., their school/company values their physical and mental health, the benefits of early identification, to improve performance). Information collected in screenings is protected health information so should not be shared without the dancer's (or in the case of minors, parent/guardian's) written consent. To protect confidentiality and maintain trusting therapeutic relationships, dancers need to know who their information will be shared with, why, and under what circumstances. Results from dancer screenings can help identify specific needs of your dancers and organization. For example, screening sessions with a dietitian might reveal that many dancers complain of small portions offered by dining services or increased dieting behaviors are being reported in a particular level in the school. Sharing de-identified data gleaned from screenings with school/company leadership allows current issues to be addressed and can help inform future prevention efforts.

If instituting a formal screening program is not feasible in your dance setting, teachers, staff, parents/caregivers, healthcare providers, and dancers themselves have a greater role and responsibility in prevention. Everyone involved in the training and care of dancers needs to be able to recognize the risk factors, signs, and symptoms of under-fueling, eating disorders, and disordered eating and know what to do when these issues are suspected—which brings us back to why education is such an essential part of prevention.

When Is the Right Time for Prevention?

Early, often, and consistently! We are born with an innate ability to regulate our intake. Babies cry when they are hungry and refuse food when they are full. Toddlers sometimes eat just a few bites and other times eat adult-size portions and then ask for more. By honoring these cues, parents/caregivers begin laying the foundation for dancers to become intuitive eaters who trust their bodies.[61]

Parents/caregivers can protect against dieting, disordered eating, and body dissatisfaction by teaching and modeling body acceptance and a belief system that values health and well-being above thinness. You can support dancers in developing healthy coping tools to deal with uncomfortable emotions and difficult life stressors, so they don't turn to self-injurious behaviors (e.g., eating disorders). By nurturing a peaceful, pleasurable, and neutral food environment in the home and being a positive role model with your own eating and body image, you can help dancers cultivate a nourishing and respectful relationship with food and their body from their childhood through teen years and beyond.

Primary care physicians/pediatricians have an opportunity at every visit to ensure that a dancer is growing and developing on their expected trajectory and to check for possible indicators of dietary inadequacy (e.g., delayed menarche, anemia, frequent illness or injury). Among healthcare professionals, dancers may see physical therapists, athletic trainers, and/or conditioning coaches most often. Therefore, it's particularly beneficial for these professionals, as well as any other healthcare providers (dietitians, therapists) working with dancers regularly to screen dancers at the initial visit and periodically at follow-ups. Some of the brief screening instruments (e.g., ESP, EDSA) only take a few minutes to complete—well worth the time to help prevent serious issues from developing.

Ideally, more formal pre-participation screening would occur prior to the start of each dance semester or season.[62] But really, every healthcare visit provides a chance to catch potential concerns early. Even asking a few simple questions about menstrual function, body image, injury, mood, and/or changes in eating and exercise can reveal that a dancer needs further evaluation.[34]

It's recommended that dance schools initiate developmentally appropriate education programs to address risk factors for under-fueling, eating disorders, and disordered eating beginning when dancers are around 9–11 years old.[46] Broad implementation of prevention efforts that include education and regular screening for all dancers of adolescent age (an especially high-risk time for developing eating disorders) could have a significant impact in reducing the prevalence of eating disorders/disordered eating.[43] Educational sessions should be offered a few times a year at minimum for dancers and somewhat less frequently for those involved in their training and care. And it's never too early for dance studios and companies to start building a protective and nurturing environment that supports dancers of all ages in developing healthy fueling habits and a peaceful relationship with their body.

From a dancer's first class and throughout their training, teachers focus on helping dancers develop good technique to master the art form and prevent injury. Dancers are taught proper alignment in each position and proper execution of each step. Teachers don't want dancers to develop bad habits in their training that might cause problems in the future—problems that might impact their ability to do what they love. Teachers are quick to give corrections, especially when they see a dancer doing something that compromises their safety. Teachers and schools also address environmental factors that might contribute to injury, like shoes and flooring. We need to think about approaching the prevention of under-fueling, eating disorders, and disordered eating in the same way. Helping dancers build healthy habits and a healthy mindset is as fundamental to their success as a dancer as helping them build good technique. Every class, every rehearsal provides a new opportunity to play a part in prevention.

Main Pointes

- Everyone in a dancer's life has an important role to play in the prevention of under-fueling, eating disorders, and disordered eating.
- Family, peers, teachers/staff, and healthcare professionals can all help or hinder dancers in building healthy habits and a positive relationship with food and their body.
- The dance school/company environment is one of the most critical areas to address in prevention.
- Creating healthy, protective subcultures in dance schools and at home can benefit dancers even when they leave these safe environments.
- Education is an essential part of primary prevention which aims to prevent the development of under-fueling, eating disorders, and disordered eating.
- Secondary prevention focuses on early identification of these issues to allow for prompt intervention and prevent progression to more serious stages. Screening is a key component of secondary prevention.
- Educational sessions for dancers should target restrictive eating/inadequate fueling and body dissatisfaction (among other topics).
- All teachers and support staff should receive education on eating disorders/disordered eating and guidance on what to do and not do when concerned about a dancer.
- Any healthcare professional working with dancers needs at least basic education on eating disorders.
- Selecting the right person(s) to provide education to your dancers is critical to ensure that content is presented in a way that is helpful rather than harmful.

Notes

What are some of the barriers to prevention that you have encountered? What might help reduce these barriers?

Endnotes

* aka inadequate nutrition/fueling, energy deficiency, low energy availability, Relative Energy Deficiency in Sport (RED-S).
† e.g., the stereotype that only skinny, White, affluent girls have eating disorders (aka SWAG stereotype).[4]
‡ Male dancers were included in the study, but because of the small number of male participants, they were not included in the data analysis.[15]
§ Some risk factors (e.g., body dissatisfaction) can fall under more than one of these categories.
** Professionals with the equivalent credentials/qualifications may have a different title in other countries.
†† Some tools might be more or less appropriate for use depending on the age of the dancer.

References

1. Marques L, Alegria M, Becker AE, et al. Comparative prevalence, correlates of impairment, and service utilization for eating disorders across US ethnic groups: Implications for reducing ethnic disparities in health care access for eating disorders. *Int J Eat Disord.* 2011;44(5):412–420. doi:10.1002/eat.20787
2. Becker AE, Franko DL, Speck A, Herzog DB. Ethnicity and differential access to care for eating disorder symptoms. *Int J Eat Disord.* 2003;33(2):205–212. doi:10.1002/eat.10129
3. Nagata JM, Garber AK, Tabler JL, Murray SB, Bibbins-Domingo K. Prevalence and correlates of disordered eating behaviors among young adults with overweight or obesity. *J Gen Intern Med.* 2018;33(8):1337–1343. doi:10.1007/s11606-018-4465-z
4. Sonneville KR, Lipson SK. Disparities in eating disorder diagnosis and treatment according to weight status, race/ethnicity, socioeconomic background, and sex among college students. *Int J Eat Disord.* 2018;51(6):518–526. doi:10.1002/eat.22846
5. Swanson SA, Crow SJ, Le Grange D, Swendsen J, Merikangas KR. Prevalence and correlates of eating disorders in adolescents. Results from the national comorbidity survey replication adolescent supplement. *Arch Gen Psychiatry.* 2011;68(7):714–723. doi:10.1001/archgenpsychiatry.2011.22
6. Mountjoy M, Sundgot-Borgen J, Burke L, et al. The IOC consensus statement: Beyond the Female Athlete Triad–Relative Energy Deficiency in Sport (RED-S). *Br J Sports Med.* 2014;48(7):491–497. doi:10.1136/bjsports-2014-093502
7. Prus D, Mijatovic D, Hadzic V, et al. (Low) energy availability and its association with injury occurrence in competitive dance: Cross-sectional analysis in female dancers. *Medicina (Kaunas).* 2022;58(7). doi:10.3390/medicina58070853
8. Thomas JJ, Keel PK, Heatherton TF. Disordered eating and injuries among adolescent ballet dancers. *Eat Weight Disord.* 2011;16(3):e216–e222. doi:10.1007/BF03325136

9. Ojofeitimi S, Bronner S. Injuries in a modern dance company effect of comprehensive management on injury incidence and cost. *J Dance Med Sci.* 2011;15(3):116–122.
10. Currie A. Sport and eating disorders – Understanding and managing the risks. *Asian J Sports Med.* 2010;1(2):63–68. doi:10.5812/asjsm.34864
11. Doyle-Lucas AF, Davy BM. Development and evaluation of an educational intervention program for pre-professional adolescent ballet dancers: Nutrition for optimal performance. *J Dance Med Sci.* 2011;15(2):65–75.
12. Yannakoulia M, Sitara M, Matalas A-L. Reported eating behavior and attitudes improvement after a nutrition intervention program in a group of young female dancers. *Int J Sport Nutr Exerc Metab.* 2002;12(1):24–32. doi:10.1123/ijsnem.12.1.24
13. Torres-McGehee TM, Green JM, Leaver-Dunn D, Leeper JD, Bishop PA, Richardson MT. Attitude and knowledge changes in collegiate dancers following a short-term, team-centered prevention program on eating disorders. *Percept Mot Skills.* 2011;112(3):711–725. doi:10.2466/06.PMS.112.3.711-725
14. Mathisen TF, Sundgot-Borgen C, Anstensrud B, Sundgot-Borgen J. Intervention in professional dance students to increase mental health- and nutrition literacy: A controlled trial with follow up. *Front Sports Act Living.* 2022;4:727048. doi:10.3389/fspor.2022.727048
15. Piran N. Eating disorders: A trial of prevention in a high risk school setting. *J Prim Prev.* 1999;20:75–90.
16. Gorrell S, Schaumberg K, Boswell JF, Hormes JM, Anderson DA. Female athlete body project intervention with professional dancers: A pilot trial. *Eat Disord.* 2021;29(1):56–73. doi:10.1080/10640266.2019.1632592
17. Bar RJ, Cassin SE, Dionne MM. The long-term impact of an eating disorder prevention program for professional ballet school students: A 15-year follow-up study. *Eat Disord.* 2017;25(5):375–387. doi:10.1080/10640266.2017.130873 1
18. Martinsen M, Bahr R, Børresen R, Holme I, Pensgaard AM, Sundgot-Borgen J. Preventing eating disorders among young elite athletes: A randomized controlled trial. *Med Sci Sports Exerc.* 2014;46(3):435–447. doi:10.1249/MSS.0b013e3182a702fc
19. Berge JM, Winkler MR, Larson N, Miller J, Haynos AF, Neumark-Sztainer D. Intergenerational transmission of parent encouragement to diet from adolescence into adulthood. *Pediatrics.* 2018;141(4). doi:10.1542/peds.2017-2955
20. Doria N, Numer M. Dancing in a culture of disordered eating: A feminist poststructural analysis of body and body image among young girls in the world of dance. *PLoS ONE.* 2022;17(1):e0247651. doi:10.1371/journal.pone.0247651
21. Tylka TL, Annunziato RA, Burgard D, et al. The weight-inclusive versus weight-normative approach to health: Evaluating the evidence for prioritizing well-being over weight loss. *J Obes.* 2014;2014:983495. doi:10.1155/2014/983495
22. Toro J, Guerrero M, Sentis J, Castro J, Puértolas C. Eating disorders in ballet dancing students: Problems and risk factors. *Eur Eat Disord Rev.* 2009;17(1):40–49. doi:10.1002/erv.888
23. Annus A, Smith GT. Learning experiences in dance class predict adult eating disturbance. *Eur Eat Disord Rev.* 2009;17(1):50–60. doi:10.1002/erv.899
24. Francisco R, Alarcão M, Narciso I. Aesthetic sports as high-risk contexts for eating disorders–Young elite dancers and gymnasts perspectives. *Span J Psychol.* 2012;15(1):265–274. doi:10.5209/rev_sjop.2012.v15.n1.37333

25. Dantas AG, Alonso DA, Sánchez-Miguel PA, Del Río Sánchez C. Factors dancers associate with their body dissatisfaction. *Body Image*. 2018;25:40–47. doi:10.1016/j.bodyim.2018.02.003

26. Reel JJ, Jamieson KM, SooHoo S, Gill DL. Femininity to the extreme: Body image concerns among college female dancers. *Women Sport Phys Act J*. 2005;14(1):39–51. doi:10.1123/wspaj.14.1.39

27. Tosi M, Maslyanskaya S, Dodson NA, Coupey SM. The female athlete triad: A comparison of knowledge and risk in adolescent and young adult figure skaters, dancers, and runners. *J Pediatr Adolesc Gynecol*. 2019;32(2):165–169. doi:10.1016/j.jpag.2018.10.007

28. Thompson RA, Sherman R. Reflections on athletes and eating disorders. *Psychol Sport Exerc*. 2014;15(6):729–734. doi:10.1016/j.psychsport.2014.06.005

29. Biesecker AC, Martz DM. Impact of coaching style on vulnerability for eating disorders: An analog study. *Eat Disord*. 1999;7(3):235–244. doi:10.1080/10640269908249289

30. Mainwaring L, Krasnow D. Teaching the dance class: Strategies to enhance skill acquisition, mastery and positive self-image. *J Dance Educ*. 2010;10(1):14–21. doi:10.1080/15290824.2010.10387153

31. Bar RJ, Cassin SE, Dionne MM. Eating disorder prevention initiatives for athletes: A review. *Eur J Sport Sci*. 2016;16(3):325–335. doi:10.1080/1746139 1.2015.1013995

32. Bratland-Sanda S, Sundgot-Borgen J. Eating disorders in athletes: Overview of prevalence, risk factors and recommendations for prevention and treatment. *Eur J Sport Sci*. 2013;13(5):499–508. doi:10.1080/17461391.2012.740504

33. Hood MM, Corsica JA. Eating disorders in adolescence: When should prevention occur? *J Am Diet Assoc*. 2011;111(7):1001–1003. doi:10.1016/j. jada.2011.04.013

34. Coelho GM de O, Gomes AI da S, Ribeiro BG, Soares E de A. Prevention of eating disorders in female athletes. *Open Access J Sports Med*. 2014;5:105–113. doi:10.2147/OAJSM.S36528

35. Wyon MA, Hutchings KM, Wells A, Nevill AM. Body mass index, nutritional knowledge, and eating behaviors in elite student and professional ballet dancers. *Clin J Sport Med*. 2014;24(5):390–396. doi:10.1097/JSM.0000000000000054

36. National Eating Disorders Collaboration (NEDC). Eating disorders in schools: Prevention, early identification and response. Second Edition. Published online 2016. Accessed January 14, 2023. https://nedc.com.au/assets/NEDC-Resources /NEDC-Resource-Schools.pdf

37. Gumz A, Weigel A, Daubmann A, Wegscheider K, Romer G, Löwe B. Efficacy of a prevention program for eating disorders in schools: A cluster-randomized controlled trial. *BMC Psychiatry*. 2017;17(1):293. doi:10.1186/ s12888-017-1454-4

38. Ranby KW, Aiken LS, Mackinnon DP, et al. A mediation analysis of the ATHENA intervention for female athletes: Prevention of athletic-enhancing substance use and unhealthy weight loss behaviors. *J Pediatr Psychol*. 2009;34(10):1069–1083. doi:10.1093/jpepsy/jsp025

39. O'dea J. School-based interventions to prevent eating problems: First do no harm. *Eat Disord*. 2000;8(2):123–130. doi:10.1080/10640260008251219

40. National Eating Disorders Association (NEDA). Giving safe presentations on eating disorders. Accessed January 22, 2023. https://www.nationaleatingd isorders.org/sites/default/files/GivingSafePresentationsFINAL.pdf

41. Doley JR, Hart LM, Stukas AA, Morgan AJ, Rowlands DL, Paxton SJ. Development of guidelines for giving community presentations about eating disorders: A Delphi study. *J Eat Disord*. 2017;5:54. doi:10.1186/ s40337-017-0183-x

42. Doley JR, Hart LM, Stukas AA, Morgan AJ, Rowlands DL, Paxton SJ. Development of guidelines for giving community presentations about eating disorders: A Delphi study. Supplementary material 1. Table 1 Items endorsed in round one by scale and panel group. *J Eat Disord.* 2017;5:54.

43. Stice E, Marti CN, Shaw H, Rohde P. Meta-analytic review of dissonance-based eating disorder prevention programs: Intervention, participant, and facilitator features that predict larger effects. *Clin Psychol Rev.* 2019;70:91–107. doi:10.1016/j.cpr.2019.04.004

44. Columbia Center for Teaching and Learning (CTL). Learning through discussion. Accessed January 22, 2023. https://ctl.columbia.edu/resources-and-technology/resources/learning-through-discussion/

45. Wells KR, Jeacocke NA, Appaneal R, et al. The Australian Institute of Sport (AIS) and National Eating Disorders Collaboration (NEDC) position statement on disordered eating in high performance sport. *Br J Sports Med.* 2020;54(21):1247–1258. doi:10.1136/bjsports-2019-101813

46. Sundgot-Borgen J, Meyer NL, Lohman TG, et al. How to minimise the health risks to athletes who compete in weight-sensitive sports review and position statement on behalf of the Ad Hoc Research Working Group on Body Composition, Health and Performance, under the auspices of the IOC Medical Commission. *Br J Sports Med.* 2013;47(16):1012–1022. doi:10.1136/bjsports-2013-092966

47. Stice E, Shaw H, Marti CN. A meta-analytic review of eating disorder prevention programs: Encouraging findings. *Annu Rev Clin Psychol.* 2007;3:207–231. doi:10.1146/annurev.clinpsy.3.022806.091447

48. Meneses C, Istifo N, Lombamo G. Large group teaching. Accessed January 23, 2023. https://openpress.usask.ca/instructionalstrategiesinhpe/chapter/large-group-teaching/

49. The Victorian Centre of Excellence in Eating Disorders and the Eating Disorders Foundation of Victoria. An Eating Disorders Resource for Schools. A manual to promote early intervention and prevention of eating disorders in schools. Published online 2004. Accessed January 23, 2023. https://nedc.com.au/assets/Uploads/Resource.-for-Schools.-An-Eating-Disorders.-A-manual-to-promote-early-intervention-and-prevention-of-eating-disorders-in-schools.pdf

50. Academy of Nutrition and Dietetics. About RDNs and NDTRs. Accessed January 24, 2023. https://www.eatright.org/about-rdns-and-ndtrs

51. Peterson TJ. Types of mental health professionals: Education, credentials, licenses & more. April 22, 2020. Accessed January 24, 2023. https://www.choosingtherapy.com/types-of-mental-health-professionals/

52. Gideon N, Hawkes N, Mond J, Saunders R, Tchanturia K, Serpell L. Development and psychometric validation of the EDE-QS, a 12 item short form of the Eating Disorder Examination Questionnaire (EDE-Q). *PLoS ONE.* 2016;11(5):e0152744. doi:10.1371/journal.pone.0152744

53. Hazzard VM, Schaefer LM, Mankowski A, et al. Development and validation of the Eating Disorders Screen for Athletes (EDSA): A brief screening tool for male and female athletes. *Psychol Sport Exerc.* 2020;50. doi:10.1016/j.psychsport.2020.101745

54. Cotton M-A, Ball C, Robinson P. Four simple questions can help screen for eating disorders. *J Gen Intern Med.* 2003;18(1):53–56. doi:10.1046/j.1525-1497.2003.20374.x

55. Perry L, Morgan J, Reid F, et al. Screening for symptoms of eating disorders: Reliability of the SCOFF screening tool with written compared to oral delivery. *Int J Eat Disord.* 2002;32(4):466–472. doi:10.1002/eat.10093

56. Bryant E, Miskovic-Wheatley J, Touyz SW, Crosby RD, Koreshe E, Maguire S. Identification of high risk and early stage eating disorders: First validation of a digital screening tool. *J Eat Disord.* 2021;9(1):109. doi:10.1186/s40337-021-00464-y

57. Hamilton L, Solomon R, Solomon J. A proposal for standardized psychological screening of dancers. *J Dance Med Sci.* 2006;10:40–45.

58. EDSA. Eating Disorders Screen for Athletes. Frequently asked questions. Accessed January 24, 2023. https://sites.google.com/view/edsa-screening-tool/faq

59. Keay N, Overseas A, Francis G. Indicators and correlates of low energy availability in male and female dancers. *BMJ Open Sport Exerc Med.* 2020;6(1):e000906. doi:10.1136/bmjsem-2020-000906

60. Melin A, Tornberg AB, Skouby S, et al. The LEAF questionnaire: A screening tool for the identification of female athletes at risk for the female athlete triad. *Br J Sports Med.* 2014;48(7):540–545. doi:10.1136/bjsports-2013-093240

61. Ellyn Satter Institute. Raise a healthy child who is a joy to feed. Follow the Satter Division of Responsibility in Feeding. Accessed January 25, 2023. https://www.ellynsatterinstitute.org/how-to-feed/the-division-of-responsibility-in-feeding/

62. Healthy Dancer Canada – The Dance Health Alliance of Canada. Dancer screening. Information for Dancers, Dance Educators and Healthcare Professionals. Published online 2019. Accessed January 23, 2023. https://www.healthydancercanada.org/uploads/4/7/1/3/47130231/hdc_dancerscreening_rp_2019.pdf

5 Prevention: Language, Messages, and Modeling

When a flower doesn't bloom you fix the environment in which it grows, not the flower.
~Alexander den Heijer

I recently presented a workshop on the importance of language—specifically, how we can shift the way we speak about food and bodies to help prevent eating disorders and improve dancer health and well-being. One of the audience members courageously shared how, beginning at eight years old, she was repeatedly told by her dance teachers that her thighs were too big for her to be a dancer. As she spoke 30 plus years later, this memory still brought her to tears.

One of my adult dancer clients described what birthday celebrations in her studio were like when she was a young adolescent. Their director would pull a slice of cake out of a dancer's hands and say, "you're too fat to eat cake." Years later, and even though my client's own piece was never taken away, these images come flooding back when she is around desserts and cause feelings of intense shame and guilt. She is still working to heal from the way this experience linked her body image to feeling she has permission to eat.

These are just two examples among countless others I have heard over the years from current and former dancers. And those stories are just the ones that have been shared with me—imagine how many others there are. Too many painful experiences of body shaming and encouragement of disordered eating that profoundly affect how dancers feel about, nourish, and care for themselves—in many cases, long after they've stopped dancing.

How Can We Protect Dancers?

How can we prevent dancers from enduring this harm? How can we reduce dancers' exposure to messages and influences like these that negatively impact their physical and mental health? How can we instead increase positive forces in dancers' environments that will help them develop a healthy relationship with food, their body, and themselves?

DOI: 10.4324/9781003366171-7

First, we must recognize that what we communicate to dancers can have a profound and lasting impact. Words hurt and language matters, as do the other messages sent to dancers through the choices, actions, and inactions of those who train and care for them. Dancers are affected by what they hear and see all around them—in their family, in the dance world, in healthcare settings, and in society, as well as by the language they use to speak to themselves.

We need to evaluate our language and messaging to ensure we are not exacerbating risk factors for under-fueling, eating disorders, and disordered eating in dancers. What language, messages, and practices might reinforce the thin ideal, contribute to body dissatisfaction, or encourage dieting, restrictive eating, and harmful weight control behaviors? What are dancers seeing and hearing that might adversely shape how they feel about food, eating, and their body? What factors in a dancer's environment might be barriers to practicing self-care or developing a strong sense of self-worth? Once we become aware of the potentially harmful language and messages dancers are exposed to, we can begin to shift what we say and do to help improve their health and well-being.

As described in Chapter 4 (see Figure 4.1), we can think of prevention in terms of aiming to tip the balance away from harmful beliefs and behaviors toward healthy habits and a healthy mindset. While we work together to reduce and eliminate modifiable risk factors for under-fueling, eating disorders, and disordered eating, we also need to focus on increasing protective factors that can decrease the likelihood of dancers developing these issues. Table 5.1 lists some of these protective factors, most of which can be reinforced in multiple domains (e.g., the dance studio, home, healthcare settings).

Table 5.1 Protective Factors

Healthy and peaceful relationship with food
Body neutrality, respect, acceptance, and/or appreciation
Appreciation of body diversity
Environment, family, and peer groups that do not over-emphasize body size/shape, weight, or appearance
Supportive relationships with family and friends
Healthy coping tools
High self-esteem and self-worth
Practicing self-care and responding to body cues (e.g., hunger, need for rest)
Self-compassion
Positive self-talk
Media literacy

Adapted from Levine and Smolak[1] and the National Eating Disorders Collaboration.[2]

The impact of protective factors tends to be related and cumulative.[1] In other words, the more a dancer is exposed to protective influences, the more those messages are reinforced and the greater the benefit. Our goal should be immersive prevention.

This chapter focuses on how we can use language, messaging, and modeling to decrease risk factors and increase protective factors to prevent dancers from developing issues that compromise their physical and mental health and performance.

A Pause for Self-Compassion

Before we delve into the discussion of language and messaging, let's take a self-compassion pause. As covered in Chapter 1, the influence of diet culture is powerful, far-reaching, and amplified in the dance world. Some of the information and recommendations you encounter here may be new to you. They might shake the foundation of diet and dance culture beliefs and practices to which you have become accustomed. There's a good chance you will read something that makes you realize you inadvertently caused harm even though that was not your intention. You might wish you could go back in time and say and do things differently. I encourage you to show yourself grace and compassion as you make space for this discomfort that is part of being human. Be kind to yourself while you're on this journey of unlearning and relearning—it will help you stay open and motivated to make the changes that are so needed in the dance world.

Language and Messages Matter

You look so much better. I don't know what you're doing to lose weight but keep up the good work.

Suck in those stomachs. I can see what you had for lunch!

It's time to lay off the junk food to get in shape for the performance.

You're a beautiful dancer but we want you to lose some weight. Don't do anything crazy. Just a few pounds.

Look at how thick your legs look in these photos. You're eating too many carbs.

Your weight is normal. Labs look fine. I don't think you have an eating disorder.

What did you think reading these statements? How did they make you feel? Have you heard or said similar things? Maybe you've heard sentiments like these so often you've become numb to them. Or perhaps these statements remind you of pain you experienced when they were said to you.

These examples were all recently said to dancer clients of mine by teachers, a choreographer, an artistic director, a parent, and a doctor. And sadly, I've been hearing versions of these statements for decades—from the time I was a dancer to the present. In my work with dancers, I see how experiences like these can impact their physical and mental health. For example, although one comment alone does not cause an eating disorder, in the context of other predisposing factors, it may be the event that "pulls the trigger."[3-5] Qualitative research[4,6-8] provides additional insight into how dancers are affected by the language and messages that they are exposed to. Consider what dancers shared in some of these studies:

"I have hips. I have breasts. ... All the things that a woman has. It makes me often think about the idea that I heard about the ideal dancer's body being one that is prepubescent so that it tries to break away from that womanhood. It goes for that muscular, lean look—no curves, nothing. That idea pops into my head so often."[7]

"I think it's a problem that is going to follow me all my life, like many dancers. It just doesn't go away when you stop dancing. ... Sometimes I am so ashamed of being fat, I can't take it anymore. You know sometimes it just comes back to haunt me and then I say to myself: 'ok, it's over, it's over.'"[4]

"There are always students who must lose weight, who don't have the 'body.' ... There are others who will lose weight even if they're not asked to lose weight. The result: 'Wow, have you seen Marie? She's been transformed, her lines are great. Marie, your lines are great, your work is great and you're moving so well.' She did nothing but lose weight."[4]

"I had a close friend that had an extreme eating disorder ... She was being held up as an exemplar. ... Constantly has solos in concerts, is presented as this person to look up to. But never in the light of 'be careful of your body.' That was never mentioned. ... I'm not sure why that is, especially in a dance department, that it's not discussed openly ... I feel like the teachers don't discuss this much. If anything, they tell you, 'You need to lose weight.'"[8]

"Sean ... described a painful experience in a New York dance studio locker room in which he was feminized by a more muscular male dancer who mocked him for carrying extra body fat. The dancer teased him about his soft looking thighs and lack of defined abs. He warned Sean that he should lose weight if he wanted to dance in a company."[8]

Different studies, genres, and dancers, but similar themes. These quotes highlight the profound impact of verbal and non-verbal messages dancers receive. As mentioned in the Prologue, I don't believe that the vast majority of people who train and care for dancers intend to cause harm. Rather, I think there is a lack of understanding about how harmful certain language and messaging can be, particularly because much of it has been passed down from generation to generation in diet culture, in the dance world, in families, and in the training of healthcare professionals. It's time to change that tradition. We can no longer say and do things just because that's what's been said and done in the past.

Standard Precautions

When I speak with parents, dance educators, and healthcare professionals about the importance of language, many report they are more careful with what they say if a dancer has an eating disorder. But how could you possibly identify every dancer with an eating disorder? And what about dancers who are at higher risk for developing eating disorders, disordered eating, and under-fueling but the issues have not yet emerged? How will you be able to identify these vulnerable dancers to modify your language accordingly? For example, female dancers with higher levels of perfectionism appear to be more susceptible to messages and practices in the dance setting that reinforce the thin ideal such as diet and weight talk from teachers and peers, weight checks, and observing restrictive eating (e.g., they are more likely to internalize the belief that restricting food intake and losing weight will be beneficial to them as dancers).[9]

So, although it is critical to be sensitive to what and how we communicate with dancers with eating disorders, our efforts cannot stop there. Eating disorders and disordered eating are often challenging to detect and the risk factors that contribute to them (e.g., body dissatisfaction, perfectionism) are even harder to see. As discussed in Chapter 3, you cannot tell whether a dancer has an eating disorder, or the severity of the eating disorder, based on their appearance.* You will not be able to identify every dancer at risk for or already engaging in harmful behaviors. More importantly, we should protect all dancers, not just those we view as most vulnerable.

If you've ever worked in a healthcare facility, you're probably familiar with standard precautions, the safety measures (e.g., handwashing, wearing gloves) taken to prevent the spread of infection. You don't always know which patients are contagious, so you use precautions with everyone. We need to apply a similar approach to the precautions we take to prevent eating disorders, disordered eating, and under-fueling in dancers—using standard precautions universally. We need to carefully consider what we do and say around every dancer. We need to apply the same sensitivity we would use if we knew a dancer had an eating disorder to all our interactions with all dancers.

Our explicit and implicit language and messaging about food, eating, weight, and bodies is particularly important to evaluate. We need to speak about these topics in a way that helps dancers develop nourishing fueling habits and a healthy relationship with food, encourages body acceptance, cultivates self-worth, and helps manage unhealthy perfectionism. We need to shift what we do and say to support dancers in developing healthy beliefs and behaviors that can serve as a shield when they encounter negative influences in the dance world and in society. By doing so we can help prevent dancers from developing eating disorders, disordered eating, and under-fueling, and we can promote and support recovery in dancers who are already dealing with these issues.

The next three sections contain guidelines for language and messaging regarding food/eating, weight, and bodies. Messaging is most beneficial when it is repeated, consistent,[10] and reinforced in multiple settings. Therefore, these guidelines are important for everyone involved in the training and care of dancers—parents, teachers, staff, peers, and healthcare professionals—to adopt and to use with all dancers.

These recommendations are presented as practical don'ts and dos, along with their rationale. I don't typically find dichotomous approaches to be the most useful. However, in these areas, I believe strongly that the don'ts should be avoided because of harm that they are likely to cause, and I support universal implementation of the dos because of their potential to provide a meaningful protective benefit.

Language and Messages Matter: Food/Eating

The language and messaging guidelines below will help dancers nourish their body and develop a peaceful and healthy relationship with food. These recommendations are intended to decrease risk factors and increase protective factors related to food and eating as shown in Figure 5.1.

Don't Encourage or Support Dieting

Given the well-documented dangers of dieting and the strong link between dieting and eating disorder development (see Chapter 1), one of the most beneficial things we can do to protect dancers' health is to prevent them from dieting. Keep in mind that even diets that are (sneakily) presented as "healthy" lifestyle changes are likely to be harmful.

Don't encourage dancers to diet or suggest other restrictive eating practices (e.g., eliminating food groups, cutting portion sizes). If a dancer asks or tells you about a diet they are considering, it's helpful to inquire about what they are hoping the diet will help them achieve (e.g., to lose weight, feel better, improve health) and to remind them of the multitude of negative health and performance consequences linked to dieting.

Don't Engage In or Allow "Diet Talk"

Diet talk refers to conversations or comments about diets or restricted eating, usually for the purpose of changing body size or shape, though occasionally diets are undertaken to "detox" or "reset."

Risk Factors

- Dieting
- Restrictive eating
- Negative energy balance
- Food rules & rigidity
- Comparison

Protective Factors

- Meet nutrient needs
- Balanced & consistent intake
- Food neutrality
- Food variety & flexibility
- Trust & listen to body cues
- Honor unique needs

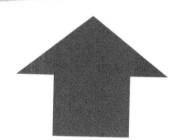

Figure 5.1 Decreasing Risk Factors and Increasing Protective Factors Related to Food and Eating.

Diet talk might sound like, "I can't eat that. I'm trying to be good" or "Cutting out carbs helped me lose weight" or "I ate so much at lunch. No dinner for me" or "I only eat whole foods, nothing processed." Diet talk may perpetuate the idea that body size earns your permission to eat—"You're so lucky you can eat that. You're so skinny!"

Diet talk is so normalized in our society that we often don't realize we are being exposed to it, participating in it, or how detrimental it can be. Diet talk can introduce dancers to harmful weight control behaviors they were previously unaware of, and it normalizes, encourages, and spreads dieting behaviors (i.e., the "contagion" effect[11] discussed in Chapter 4). Diet talk also contributes to comparison. A dancer may think, "If they don't eat x, I shouldn't either" or "If they think that was a big portion, what must they think about mine?"

It's critical to not engage in diet talk yourself, which may take practice as it may have become a habit you haven't been aware of. Don't allow your dancers to participate in diet talk either. If you hear diet talk, you can shut it down by saying "This is a diet-talk free zone!" Additional strategies to counter diet talk are provided in Table 5.3.

Don't Label Foods as Good/Bad

This dichotomous approach to food is inaccurate and is particularly problematic for dancers who are often perfectionists and may be prone to black-and-white thinking. Categorizing foods as good/bad or healthy/unhealthy doesn't account for individual needs or acknowledge how socioeconomic status, culture, and other factors contribute to food choice and health. For example, vegetables are often considered "good," and dancers may be encouraged to increase their intake of this "healthy" food group. But for some dancers, such as those with certain digestive issues or recovering from an eating disorder, eating more vegetables may not be a healthy choice.

Labeling foods as good/bad reinforces the diet culture message that food choices are a reflection of our morality. Consequently, dancers may judge themselves for being a good or bad person based on what they eat/don't eat. When dancers believe that a food they ate is "bad" or "unhealthy" (or that they are bad for eating it), they might have an increased desire to compensate by engaging in harmful behaviors. This rigid way of viewing food can make eating a source of stress, fear, and anxiety[12]—far more problematic for a dancer's health than any one food could be.

Nutrition occurs on a spectrum and food is meant to be both nourishing and enjoyable. There are no inherently "bad" or "unhealthy" foods, except perhaps those that are spoiled or that a dancer is allergic to.

Don't Use Judgmental Language to Describe Food/Eating

To help dancers develop a neutral and peaceful relationship with food, it's important to avoid language that assigns value to food or makes dancers feel judged for what, how much, or how they are eating. Consider what message you are sending by calling food "junk," a "splurge," or even a "treat" (vs. referring to it in a more neutral way by calling it what it is— pizza, a cookie, etc.). Refrain from making comments about the quantity of food a dancer is consuming or their pace of eating such as, "You must be starving. You inhaled that!" or "That's a lot of carbs!" or "Is today your cheat day?" Even comments that might be intended as a compliment, for example, praising a dancer for their self-restraint if they only eat a small portion of dessert, can be harmful (you might be applauding an eating disorder behavior).

Don't Promote a Compensatory Approach to Eating

Dancers should not be encouraged to save up or make up for specific foods or amounts that they eat (e.g., saving up for holiday meals by skipping meals/snacks or making up for a "bad" food choice by doing extra exercise or deliberately decreasing intake at the next meal/snack). Although this approach is often viewed as self-discipline, it is a disordered eating behavior. Intentional compensation is different than honoring your body's cues. For example, after having a rich meal, you might feel less hungry at your next meal/snack and intuitively adjust how much you eat (or you might feel just as hungry or hungrier and it's important to respect these body signals too).

Don't Give Out Nutrition Information without Considering the Impact

Even ostensibly benign nutrition recommendations like "eat more whole grains" can be potentially problematic. It's critical that anyone providing dancers with nutrition information is adequately qualified to do so, experienced in evaluating the potential impact of their message, and skilled at presenting nutrition concepts in a way that does not cause harm. Qualified nutrition professionals (i.e., Registered Dietitians) must also carefully consider how nutrition education is delivered to dancers and the explicit and implicit messages they may be sending (e.g., don't show pictures of meals with very small portions or give general nutrition recommendations such as "fill half your plate with veggies").

A part of human nature is wanting to share things we find helpful with people we care about. However, avoid sharing nutrition strategies that "worked" for you (e.g., "I feel so much less bloated after I cut out carbs at dinner"). Although you might not be suggesting that the dancer use the same strategy, they are likely to take it that way and/or compare their eating habits to yours. On the other hand, it might be helpful for dancers to hear that you found working with a therapist or dietitian beneficial because it normalizes seeking support from qualified professionals.

Do Promote an All Foods Fit Approach

Although different foods offer varying types and amounts of nutrients, almost everything we consume is made of carbohydrates, protein, and/or fat, and therefore has nutrient value. In addition, providing nutrients is not the only function of food. Food is more than just fuel—it is pleasure, connection, celebration, culture, and more. Dancers don't need to limit their food intake to just items that have maximum nutritional value. It is normal and appropriate to eat for other reasons including for enjoyment, to participate in an experience, or because that food is what's available.

An all foods fit approach neither moralizes nor villainizes any food choice. This way of viewing food/eating helps counter judgment, shame, and guilt about eating certain foods and supports dancers in developing a peaceful, rather than stress-inducing, relationship with food. When dancers believe that all foods have a place in their diet, they are able to be more flexible, which also supports them in eating enough (e.g., a dancer prefers to eat whole grains because they have more fiber, but if that choice isn't available, they are easily able to eat a refined grain option instead).

Do Teach Dancers to Tune in to Their Body's Wisdom

All foods can fit, but that doesn't mean that every food choice will serve a dancer in every situation. For example, there's nothing wrong with eating a candy bar, but how does a dancer feel when they eat this before a three-hour rehearsal? Does it help them have sustained energy and feel and dance their best?

Rather than using an external set of rules about what, when, and how much to eat, we can teach dancers how to tune in to their body's wisdom to guide their food choices. This approach helps dancers build body trust and practice self-care. Instead of judging or ignoring body signals that let them know when food (or rest or comfort) is needed and how much, they appreciate and honor these messages.

Sometimes honoring your body means knowing when your hunger and fullness cues aren't accurate and eating anyway because your body needs fuel (e.g., when intense dancing or heightened emotions decrease appetite or if hunger cues are suppressed because a dancer has been under-fueling). Honoring your body also means eating in a way that supports performance and recovery. For example, dancers often need to eat during breaks (that don't necessarily line up with when they are hungry) because waiting would lead to dancing in an energy-deficient state. We want to help dancers learn when to use their body cues and when to eat strategically.

Do Be Very Cautious with Numbers-Based Nutrition

Numbers-based approaches to eating are not practical or healthy. Discussing food and eating in terms of calories, grams of sugar, grams of fat, macronutrient percentages, etc. can interfere with dancers developing a healthy and trusting relationship with food. Thinking of food in these terms can be especially problematic in the context of perfectionism and/or rigid thinking.

Tracking calories and nutrients is often harmful for dancers as this practice can lead to obsessive food thoughts and disordered eating behaviors. In addition, calorie/nutrient counting teaches dancers to make food decisions based on external factors (e.g., numerical targets) rather than listening to their body. Dancers should not be encouraged to use calorie counting apps as they often underestimate nutrition needs, especially in growing dancers, and can lead to or worsen restrictive eating and compensatory behaviors. Determining the amount of energy and nutrients a dancer needs to function optimally cannot be calculated with a simple math formula that doesn't account for individual factors or changing needs.

Do Consider Each Dancer's Unique Needs

Dancers have unique needs as aesthetic athletes and as individuals. What's best for one dancer won't necessarily be the same as what's best for their friends, family, or even their dancer peers. Encourage dancers to honor their own needs—i.e., fuel and care for their body in the way that they require, even if no one around them is doing the same thing.

Each dancer's needs and preferences need to be considered when providing guidance on food and eating. Nutrition recommendations should not be made in a Eurocentric, one-size-fits-all way that ignores how culture, socioeconomic status, and life circumstances affect access, options, and preferences.

Not every dancer needs to eat organic kale to be healthy. Some may not want to, and some may not be able to.

Should Dance Educators Discuss Nutrition?

Teachers, are you wondering if you should be talking to your dancers about nutrition at all? Maybe you are thinking teaching dancers how to eat well is their parents' responsibility. As a dance educator, it is neither in your scope as a teacher, nor is it helpful to give dancers nutrition advice, unless you have the necessary training to do so (i.e., you are a qualified nutrition professional). However, teachers can play a key role in helping dancers develop healthy habits and a healthy mindset.

Dancers often trust and do what teachers say without question,[6] so it's essential to avoid the harmful language/messaging discussed in this section. Ideally, parents/caregivers are teaching dancers how to fuel optimally and have a healthy relationship with food. Unfortunately, not all dancers have a family system that is able to provide this guidance. In addition, as mentioned in the last chapter, many dancers spend more time in the studio than they do at home. The dance environment can have a significant, and perhaps greater, influence than the home environment, especially for dancers training away from their families or for those lacking family support and/or stability.

Although teachers shouldn't give specific nutrition recommendations to dancers, here are some helpful things teachers can do/say to support dancers in nourishing their bodies and developing a healthy relationship with food:

• Reinforce the need to eat enough for performance and health (e.g., dancers should not skip meals/snacks).
• Remind dancers to fuel and hydrate on breaks.
• Remind dancers that diets are harmful, especially for growing dancers.
• Reinforce the idea that there are no good/bad foods, and all foods can fit.
• Stop diet talk when you hear it.
• Discourage commenting on or comparison with other people's food choices or eating habits.

Language and Messages Matter: Weight

As discussed in Chapter 1, several factors in the dance world contribute to dancers being preoccupied with weight, fearing weight gain, and feeling that their bodies are larger than "ideal." As just one example, many dancers are told to lose weight during their training and career, usually by their teachers or directors.[4,13] When dancers are afraid of gaining weight, are not happy with their weight, or feel or hear that their teachers/directors want them to lose weight, they are more likely to diet and engage in other disordered eating behaviors.[4,14,15] Multiple studies have shown that just believing that one's weight is too high (e.g., self-identifying as "overweight"[16] or "heavy"[17] or desiring weight loss[18]), regardless of whether that perception is accurate,[†] is associated with negative health consequences such as increased depression,[16] physiological dysregulation (e.g., unfavorable changes in blood pressure, blood sugar, inflammatory markers),[16] elevated levels of the stress hormone cortisol,[17] and poorer self-rated physical and mental health.[16,18]

The below guidelines address language and messaging that contribute to overconcern and dissatisfaction with weight. By eliminating the don'ts and increasing the dos, we decrease the likelihood that dancers will engage in harmful behaviors to change their weight/size and we help protect their physical and mental health. Risk and protective factors related to weight and body image are shown in Figure 5.2.

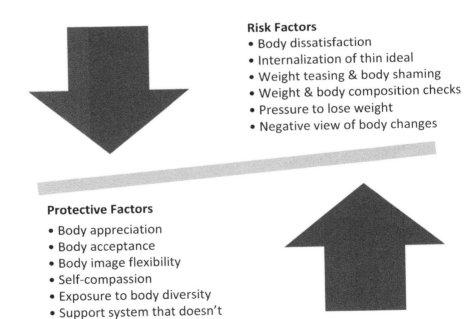

Risk Factors
- Body dissatisfaction
- Internalization of thin ideal
- Weight teasing & body shaming
- Weight & body composition checks
- Pressure to lose weight
- Negative view of body changes

Protective Factors
- Body appreciation
- Body acceptance
- Body image flexibility
- Self-compassion
- Exposure to body diversity
- Support system that doesn't over-value appearance

Figure 5.2 Decreasing Risk Factors and Increasing Protective Factors Related to Weight and Body Image.

Adapted from the National Eating Disorders Collaboration,[2] Wells et al.,[30] Levine and Smolak,[1] and Wood-Barcalow et al.[31]

Don't Encourage Weight Loss

I frequently get asked, "How can I tell a dancer they need to lose weight without damaging them?" I appreciate the awareness that there are negative consequences to telling a dancer their body is bigger than "ideal" and that teachers/directors want to avoid causing harm. And, given all the reasons just discussed, it is not possible to have this type of conversation with a dancer (aka the dreaded "fat talk") in a way that ensures harm won't be done. There are certainly ways to instruct a dancer to lose weight that are more damaging than others—explicitly body-shaming or insulting the dancer, threatening them with the loss of a role or contract, telling them to lose a specific amount of weight and/or in a short period of time, and not providing them with resources for professional help.[‡] But the only way to guarantee that you won't cause harm by telling a dancer to lose weight is to not have the discussion at all.

Saying to a dancer that you want them to tone, lengthen, or get fit does not diminish the negative impact. Most dancers know these euphemisms are code for "you need to lose weight." Attempting to change the expectation from thin to fit doesn't lessen the pressure dancers feel to achieve the "ideal" body.[6] The directive to "get fit" may also create confusion by conflating weight with fitness. Weight loss can lead to a dancer becoming less fit (e.g., they are under-fueling to lose weight, the lower weight is below where their body functions optimally). It is also not helpful to give dancers instructions in a group setting (e.g., in class or rehearsal) like "all of you need to get in performance shape," because every dancer will assume the message to lose weight is meant for them.

What about encouraging "healthy" weight loss? "Just lose a little, not too much." "Don't do anything drastic—we want you to lose weight the healthy way." As described above, dancers frequently turn to harmful behaviors to lose weight or maintain a low weight. Dancers are often over-compliant, so if you tell them to lose x pounds, they might think more is better. In addition, as discussed in Chapter 1, dieting is far more likely to lead to an eating disorder or future weight gain than sustainable or "healthy" weight loss.

So, is there a way for dancers to lose weight that doesn't harm their health? Sometimes, when a dancer focuses on better meeting their nutrition needs for health and performance while also building a healthier relationship with food (which often requires guidance from a dietitian), their weight may settle in a lower place—if it's biologically appropriate for their body. However, when dancers change their eating and/or exercise habits with the intention of losing weight, and especially when weight-loss efforts are a result of direct or perceived pressure from teachers/directors or parents, the weight loss that may result is likely to come with a cost to the dancer's physical and mental health.

Hopefully after reading this section, you are reaching the conclusion that there isn't a way to tell dancers to lose weight while also prioritizing their health and well-being. Encouraging weight loss in dancers of any age can increase their risk of developing an eating disorder or suffering from any of the multitude of health and performance consequences of under-fueling, including injury. Growing dancers in particular should never be told to lose weight as this can impact their physical development and cause significant emotional damage at a time when their body and identity are still developing.

Don't Praise Weight Loss

Congratulating and celebrating weight loss is so normalized in diet culture and in dance that we often don't realize it can be harmful. Imagine for a moment that a dancer has been skipping meals and purging and has lost weight. The dancer is told, "You look great!" or "Your lines have really improved." No one (I hope) would tell this dancer to continue engaging in eating disorder behaviors to maintain their body "improvements," but that is the message that praising weight loss sends.

Remarking on a dancer's weight loss is usually well-meaning (e.g., you might be aiming to acknowledge their hard work or compliment their appearance). Sometimes, comments are not intended to praise weight loss, yet still have this outcome. For example, you might say to a dancer "You look beautiful," because you notice they look happier or have more confidence in their dancing. But, if a dancer has lost weight and gets an appearance-based compliment, they are likely to hear the message that thinner is better.

Applauding weight loss, especially without knowledge about what behaviors or circumstances are contributing to a dancer's body change, also reinforces the belief that weight loss by any means is a good thing. A dancer may interpret this praise to mean, "We don't care how you are shrinking your body; we're just happy that you are" or "Your body size is more important than your health and well-being." The best way to prevent inadvertently sending these harmful messages or reinforcing unhealthy weight-related beliefs and behaviors is to not comment on dancers' weight, body size, or appearance. Table 5.2 provides examples of recommended language shifts related to appearance and food.

Table 5.2 Language Shifts

Don't Say	Better Alternative
You look great. Have you lost weight?	I'm so happy to see you.
She's so skinny—she looks fabulous.	I love what a good listener she is.
Wow! That's a lot of food. I wish I could eat like that.	I'm happy to see you fueling your body. *(Or preferably, don't comment at all.)*
You look so much better. Glad you've gotten over that eating disorder.	How are you?
Are you really going to eat that? It's so bad for you.	*Don't comment on anyone's food choices or eating habits.*

Don't Weigh Dancers (in Dance Settings)

Dancers should not be weighed in their dance schools/companies, nor should they be required to achieve or maintain a certain weight or body fat percentage that has been decided by their school/company, as these practices compromise dancers' health. There are times when it is beneficial to weigh dancers in healthcare settings, which may include appointments with the medical team associated with their school/company. Even in these situations, careful consideration needs to be given to how dancers are weighed to not cause harm (guidelines for weighing dancers in healthcare visits are discussed later in this chapter).

Weight should be treated as personal and confidential medical information[19] and is not appropriate to be monitored by those who train or employ dancers. In addition, dance educators and artistic staff are not healthcare professionals; therefore, they do not have the necessary training or expertise to evaluate a dancer's weight. So, what is the purpose of weighing dancers?

If you are trying to ensure that dancers are healthy enough to train and perform, remember that neither weight nor BMI alone tell you if a dancer is healthy—only a thorough evaluation by a healthcare professional can inform you about a dancer's health status. In situations when a dancer needs to be cleared to perform (e.g., for a competition, when returning from eating disorder treatment), dance educators/artistic staff are not qualified to make this determination. Dancers need to see a medical provider who can confirm if it is safe for the dancer to participate. The provider can complete a form to be shared with the dance school/company/organization that indicates "cleared to dance" and state if any modifications to full participation are needed. This form does not need to (and shouldn't) include the dancer's weight.

If the reason for weighing dancers is to check that dancers are meeting your aesthetic expectations, this can be assessed without knowing their weight. Perhaps more importantly, if a dancer's weight is being used to decide if they are suitable for your school or company, I hope reading this book is making you consider that it may be time to re-evaluate the values of your organization.

Remember that dancers of any weight/size can have an eating disorder. When there is concern about a dancer's weight (e.g., a dancer is underweight[§]; there are noticeable weight changes in either direction; they are recovering from an eating disorder), it is best practice to refer the dancer for an evaluation and monitoring by a physician and dietitian with adequate training in eating disorders and experience working with dancers.

Don't Engage In or Allow Weight-Based Teasing

Weight- and body-based teasing may be viewed by some as innocuous joking, but it can cause significant harm. A recent study found "weight teasing is strongly correlated with disordered eating in both adolescence and young adulthood regardless of ethnicity/race, socioeconomic status, or gender."[20] In addition, experiencing weight teasing is linked to body dissatisfaction,[21,22] increased dieting, and the use of unhealthy and extreme weight-loss methods (e.g., skipping meals, smoking, taking diet pills).[20] Being teased by peers or family members about weight, independent of actual weight, is also associated with low self-esteem, increased depression, and suicidal thoughts and attempts in adolescent boys and girls across racial and ethnic groups.[23] Given these risks, no one involved in the training and care of dancers should comment on or criticize the weight or body size/shape of a dancer (or anyone else for that matter) or engage in or allow any form of weight-based teasing or body shaming.

Do Consider Implicit Messages about Weight

What message is sent to a dancer when they lose weight and are rewarded (e.g., with a lead role in their dance company or with a gift from their parents)? What messages do dancers receive and internalize when they see only the thinnest dancers or those with known eating disorders complimented, favored, featured, and promoted? This is not to say that thin dancers or those with eating disorders are not deserving of these accolades. But we need to consider the impact of dancers repeatedly seeing ultra-thin bodies prized in the dance world, and in some cases, valued over dancers' health. These practices are especially problematic when dancers don't also see diversity in body types, gender identities, and race/ethnicity represented (e.g., in similar roles and positions).

Do Remember Weight Is Not Indicative of Eating Habits

You can't tell anything about a dancer's eating habits based on their weight. Although diet culture perpetuates the idea that a larger body is a sign of poor eating habits and/or overeating and that eating less will always lead to weight loss, neither is true. A dancer with a weight above what you consider "ideal" may be under-eating. Because of the effects of under-fueling on metabolism, decreasing food intake may not lead to weight loss, but will further harm the dancer's health. In addition, remember that a dancer of "normal" or higher than "ideal" weight can have a severe eating disorder, including anorexia nervosa. Consider the impact of telling this dancer to eat less.

Do Evaluate Why You Are Concerned about a Dancer's Weight

If you are concerned about a possible eating disorder or other health issue, the dancer should be referred to a medical provider for an evaluation. Are there aspects of the dancer's performance (e.g., jump height, stamina, partnering) you would like to see improved and think weight loss will help? Are there other ways you can address these issues without recommending a dancer lose weight (e.g., strength training)?

Sometimes concern about a dancer's weight is motivated by wanting to help them succeed in the dance world. You see the dancer's talent, but don't think their body matches your school or company's preferred aesthetic. Or perhaps you are training a dancer who is pursuing a particular dance dream (e.g., to dance in a certain company, to be on Broadway, etc.) and you worry their body size/shape will prevent them from reaching their goals.

Here is where we need to start asking the tough questions. Is there room in your school/company to broaden the type of body that is accepted? If not, can you help the dancer find a school/company where they are better suited, so they don't have to harm themselves trying to meet unrealistic expectations? How might your (or your organization's) weight and body biases be contributing to the narrow body ideals that prevent talented dancers from sharing their gifts with audiences and the dance world? If we all wait for the current standards and expectations to change before we begin evaluating and shifting our own practices, how will the dance world ever evolve?

Language and Messages Matter: Body Image

Body dissatisfaction is common in dancers across different genres.[8,24,25] As mentioned previously, body dissatisfaction contributes to restrictive eating and other disordered eating behaviors in dancers,[15,26] and body dissatisfaction appears to be the strongest predictor of developing an eating disorder.[27] Negative body image is also associated with other health consequences such as anxiety, depression,[26,28] and increased inflammation.[29]

The language and messaging guidelines below will help dancers develop a more peaceful, accepting, and compassionate view of and relationship with their body. These recommendations are intended to decrease risk factors and increase protective factors for eating disorders, disordered eating, and under-fueling related to body image (and weight), some of which are shown in Figure 5.2.

Don't Engage In or Allow Negative Body Talk

Negative body talk (aka weight talk or fat talk) refers to comments or conversations about the size/shape of one's own body or the bodies of others. It may sound pejorative such as "I feel so huge" or "My thighs look disgusting in this costume." Or it may sound seemingly positive, "She's lost so much weight. She looks amazing now!" and still send a negative message (i.e., thinner is better, having an eating disorder is worth it).

Like diet talk, negative body talk can be contagious. One person in a group begins criticizing their body and then the body-bashing and fat-shaming spreads. "You're not fat. I'm fat," "If you think your thighs are huge, look at mine," "Did you notice how much weight he's gained? He's really let himself go." These appearance-focused comments and conversations are harmful for multiple reasons.

Participating in or being exposed to weight talk increases comparison,[22] contributes to dancers being more critical of their bodies,[32] and reinforces the message that a small body is a valuable attribute.[33] A review study that evaluated the consequences of "fat talk" found that it is associated with depression, disordered eating, body dissatisfaction, drive for thinness, and internalization of the thin ideal.[34] In addition, using "fat" (or other words that refer to a larger body size) as an insult or as a negative descriptor perpetuates weight stigma.

It's important for dancers to know that weight/body talk harms their health and therefore won't be allowed in their home or studio. Parents, siblings, teachers, staff, and healthcare professionals should not engage in weight talk or remark on the appearance of others, even if it is well-intentioned. If you hear dancers doing this, you can remind them that we all have a role to play in creating a positive and supportive environment and part of that is not commenting on our own body size or the bodies of others. Additional strategies to deal with negative body talk (and diet talk) are shown in Table 5.3.

Don't Engage In or Allow Body Shaming

Body shaming is criticizing, mocking, and/or humiliating someone (or yourself) for supposed body faults or imperfections.[35] According to the National Association of Anorexia Nervosa and Associated Disorders (ANAD), body shaming is a type of bullying that can cause severe emotional trauma.[36] As described in the examples that opened this chapter, the harmful impacts of body shaming can last a lifetime.

Weight teasing is one form of body shaming. Body shaming may also sound like negative body talk, or it may be a disapproving comment that a person is "too skinny" or "too muscular," or a criticism unrelated to body size (e.g., about skin color, the size/shape of facial features, a disability, etc.), or it may be a practice such as public weigh-ins. Body shaming may occur face-to-face, behind someone's back, or online and on social media.

In recent years, dancers have been more open about their experiences with body shaming,[37-39] which sadly remains a common and sometimes accepted practice in the dance world. Body shaming from teachers and other individuals who dancers look up to and want to please, or who have power over their future, is especially harmful.

Table 5.3 Countering Diet Talk and Negative Body Talk

Approach	Example
Honesty	This conversation is making me feel bad about my body (or is making my eating disorder voice really loud).
Advocate	I don't think it's appropriate to talk about/shame people's bodies.
Leave the environment	I need some fresh air. I'm going outside for a walk.
Change the topic	Have you seen _____ on Netflix?
Humor	I'm on a diet from talking about diets.

Research has shown that aesthetic athletes who receive or hear disparaging body comments from coaches are significantly more likely to believe they need to lose weight, to use unhealthy weight control practices, and to report having an eating disorder than those who are not exposed to these critical comments.[40] Adopting a zero-tolerance policy for body shaming in the dance world could have a significant benefit for the health and well-being of dancers.

Don't Pathologize Normal Body Changes

Bodies are supposed to change. Bodies change due to illness, injury, pregnancy, and different life stages (e.g., puberty, menopause). We need to prepare dancers for these expected shifts and help them (and the dance world) accept them rather than pathologize them. Puberty is a time of major bodily change. In addition to significant increases in height and weight, dancers also undergo hormonal, skeletal, and body composition changes[41,42] that are all necessary to grow and develop into healthy adults.

Despite pubertal changes being an essential part of human development, teachers often view puberty as a negative event with detrimental effects for dancers' physiques, especially female dancers.[43] In females, normal pubertal changes (e.g., breast development, increased body fat) move them further away from the "ideal" dancer body whereas for males, pubertal changes (e.g., increased height and musculature) are seen as desirable.[43] Consequently, female dancers may fear pubertal (and other life-related) body changes and turn to restrictive eating and other harmful practices to try to control their body.[10]

When a prepubescent body type, which is neither realistic nor healthy to maintain into adulthood, is considered the "ideal,"[43] what message does this send about the value given to dancers' health? What might shift if the dance environment helped dancers feel comfortable with and even appreciate their changing bodies?

Do Convey the Message That All Bodies Are "Good" Bodies

Comments about which dancers do and don't have "good" dancer bodies are commonplace in the dance world. Less explicit practices, such as only using dancers with an "ideal" physique to demonstrate in class, also reinforce the same harmful message that there is only one acceptable type of dancer body. Every dancer has something special and unique to offer, and we need to help dancers recognize and appreciate their own gifts.[44]

We can help create a protective environment by shifting the focus away from body size/shape and highlighting other desirable qualities like strength, stamina, perseverance, musicality, and artistry.[44,45] We can also help dancers cultivate gratitude for their body—the body that enables them to do magnificent and meaningful things as a dancer and as a human. Focusing on and appreciating body functionality (i.e., everything the body is capable of doing) fosters more positive body image and is linked to higher psychological well-being.[31] In athletes, functionality appreciation is associated with improved confidence and performance.[46]

Do Help Dancers Practice Body Image Flexibility

Body image flexibility is the ability to experience body dissatisfaction and still engage in behaviors consistent with one's values.[47,48] For example, a dancer might feel bloated and have thoughts that their stomach is too big. This dancer can practice body image flexibility by making space for such thoughts/feelings and still choosing to eat consistently throughout the day (vs. skipping meals) keeping in line with their value of caring for their body as an athlete.[47]

Body image flexibility is associated with decreased body dissatisfaction, less disordered eating, and lower levels of psychological distress (e.g., depression, anxiety, stress).[48,49] Body image flexibility also seems to have a protective role when body dissatisfaction is present—i.e., negative body image is less likely to lead to disordered eating if an individual has high body image flexibility.[48] To support dancers in building body image flexibility, we need to reinforce the message that they are worthy of nourishment, rest, and compassion regardless of what their body looks like or how they perceive their body. By doing so, we can help dancers ride the inevitable waves of negative body thoughts and feelings and cope with self-care rather than self-harming behaviors.

Do Fight for Increased Diversity, Equity, and Inclusion in Dance

Perceived body acceptance by others supports the development of nourishing, adaptive, and flexible eating habits and positive body image.[31] In other words, helping dancers feel that their body is accepted is an integral factor in improving their health and well-being. We all need to work to challenge the overly narrow and often unhealthy body ideals that persist in the dance world. Improving diversity in dance—diversity in race, ethnicity, gender, gender expression, and body type—reinforces the message that there isn't just one type of acceptable dancer body. Representation matters as does having supportive dance environments that foster a sense of belonging. Dancers need to see and feel that they have a place in dance to believe that they have a place in dance. They need this to thrive and so does the art form.

Self-Compassion Is Healthy

Self-compassion may be the antidote to multiple risk factors that compromise dancers' physical and mental health. Studies have shown that self-compassion is associated with improved body image[50] and less disordered eating, anxiety, depression, maladaptive perfectionism, and comparison.[51] In addition, people with high levels of self-compassion are more likely to practice health-promoting behaviors such as eating well-balanced meals, getting enough sleep, and stress management.[52] So, being kind (rather than harsh) toward ourselves and others may be the best way to motivate behavior change.

According to research psychologist Dr. Kristin Neff, who has studied self-compassion extensively, focusing on improving self-compassion may be more beneficial than trying to increase self-esteem.[51] Self-esteem is an evaluation of how worthy we feel[51] or how much we like and value ourselves.[53] Self-esteem is largely reliant on our sense of accomplishment and is often based on comparing ourselves to others, which makes self-esteem prone to fluctuation.[51,53]

A dancer's self-esteem may increase when they feel they are doing well in school, in dance, or socially, but this may depend on how they judge themselves compared to others (e.g., Did they get selected for a lead role? Are they getting more attention in class than other dancers?). On the other hand, self-compassion provides a more stable sense of self-worth that is not contingent on perceived successes or failures or comparison.[51] When we have self-compassion, "we can learn to feel good about ourselves ... because we're human beings intrinsically worthy of respect."[53]

There are three overlapping components of self-compassion—self-kindness (vs. self-judgment), common humanity (vs. isolation), and mindfulness (vs. over-identification).[51] We can help dancers develop and practice self-compassion through our language, messages, and modeling. For example, instead of chastising dancers for mistakes or allowing them to be overly self-critical when they don't do a step or combination properly, we can model and encourage a compassionate approach:

Every dancer makes mistakes (common humanity) so there is no need to be so harsh with yourself (self-kindness). It's okay to feel disappointed but try not to obsess over making a mistake. How can you learn from what just happened and then let it go (mindfulness)?

Similarly, we can encourage and model self-compassion to support dancers in developing a healthy relationship with food and their body (e.g., to help them cope when they feel that they've made a "mistake" with eating or when they are having an uncomfortable body day).

Additional Recommendations by Setting

Dancers hear and see things in their environment that shape their relationship with food, their body image, and sense of self-worth. What is communicated to dancers explicitly and implicitly can help or hinder them in developing healthy habits and a healthy mindset. Ideally, efforts to prevent eating disorders, disordered eating, and under-fueling would happen everywhere that a dancer is—where they live, train, work, socialize, and more. Here we will focus on considerations for three key environments—the dance studio, a dancer's home, and healthcare settings. These recommendations are just a starting point. It's important to keep learning and adding to this list. Chapter 8 offers an in-depth discussion on helping dancers develop more balanced and resilient body image.

Dance School/Studio/Company

To support dancers in developing good fueling habits and a healthy relationship with food:

- Build enough time into dancers' schedules so they can eat. Thirty minutes is usually inadequate for meals, especially if classes and rehearsals run over. A minimum one-hour break for meals is recommended.
- Offer spaces to eat and to store and prepare food (e.g., refrigerator, microwave).
- Have snacks available for purchase (e.g., vending machine or kiosk) and, if possible, offer some free options for students in financial need.
- Make information about local food assistance resources (e.g., food pantries) available for all dancers/families.
- If you have a cafeteria or dining hall, don't label food options as healthy/unhealthy (or use a similar system like green/yellow/red light) or post calorie and nutrition information. It's preferable to make nutrition information available, for those who want it, on a website or via request rather than displaying this information directly on the menu choices.

To support dancers in developing more positive (or neutral) body image:

- Consider the use and impact of mirrors. Although mirrors can be a useful tool in training, they are a major factor in the dance environment that contributes to dancers' body dissatisfaction.[6,54,55] Mirror use can lead to increased comparison, self-consciousness, and self-criticism, and can impede technical progress.[7,56] Dance educators need to be mindful of how dancers are using the mirror and how it may be affecting their mood and behavior.[57] Reducing the use of mirrors (e.g., by covering them at times or having dancers face away from the mirror) has been suggested as a potentially helpful practice.[57,58] However, mirrors adversely impact body image in large part because their use reinforces and intensifies the negative relationship that dancers have with their body, which has been shaped by pressures and expectations in the dance environment.[6] So, it's not clear how beneficial reducing mirror use will be in decreasing body dissatisfaction,[56] unless dancers are also being trained in an environment that fosters more positive body image.[6]
- Offer flexibility in your dress code. Dancers frequently cite their "uniform" as a contributing factor for their negative body image,[6,7,55] and giving dancers some choice in their dance attire can be helpful.[6] For example, if your school requires that all dancers in a certain level wear the same color leotard, allow some flexibility in style so dancers can choose the

option they feel most comfortable in (e.g., spaghetti strap, long-sleeves, etc.). Consider having days or classes that you allow dancers to wear warm-ups, black tights, a skirt, or other options that may provide some reprieve from the body pressures of the usual "uniform."

- Carefully consider the language used when giving corrections and feedback. Don't use body shaming language (e.g., "You sound like a herd of elephants," "Suck in your stomachs," "You'd have a better fifth position if your thighs were smaller") or weight-related terms like "heavy" or "light." Do use non-weight/size-related imagery and clear guidance using anatomical terms. Don't encourage comparison with peers, especially by using only dancers with the most "ideal" bodies as examples (e.g., "Do the step more like her"). Avoid giving general, vague feedback that could be interpreted as a directive to lose weight (e.g., "You need to get in shape"). Instead, provide specific instructions on what to improve and how (e.g., "I encourage doing x to improve stamina"). All corrections and feedback should be provided in a respectful, caring, and supportive way.[59,60]

- Measurements for costumes should be done in private and kept confidential.[6] Don't measure dancers in front of their peers, say dancers' measurements aloud during costume fittings,[6] or display measurements where they can be viewed by other dancers or staff (other than costume shop staff).

- When selecting costumes, be considerate of how a costume will look on a variety of body types.[6] It can be helpful to give dancers some say in costume design when possible.[6]

- Remove scales from locker rooms, dressing areas, and gyms. Medical/ healthcare offices are the only place where scales should be kept.

To create a more positive, inclusive, and safe environment:

- Provide dressing rooms and restrooms that dancers of all genders, including non-binary dancers, feel comfortable using.

- Make sure that your dress code (e.g., required hairstyles, shoe/tights color) is inclusive and affirming for dancers of all sizes, races, ethnicities, skin tones, and genders.

- Consider the images that dancers are exposed to in your studio and in marketing. Are dancers seeing diversity in body type, race, ethnicity, and gender represented in the photos on the walls, on your social media pages, and in your marketing materials? And more importantly, is this diversity also being represented in your studio and on the stage?[61]

- Ask permission to touch students (e.g., when giving corrections). Provide training to dancers on consent, safe touch, and boundaries for partnering.[62]

- Be understanding and supportive of dancers who need to make modifications (e.g., when returning from an injury or during eating disorder recovery).

- Encourage dancers to use their voice.[6,10] When dancers share their concerns or make suggestions for constructive change, ensure they feel heard and know how the issues will be addressed.[10]

Home Environment

To help dancers develop good fueling habits and a healthy relationship with food:

- Reinforce the importance of consistent, balanced, and adequate nourishment and provide meals and snacks in a way that supports this. (See Chapter 6 for more specific nutrition guidance. Additional resources for parents are provided in the Appendix.)
- Offer and speak about foods in a neutral way. Make a variety of choices available and accessible on a regular basis, including foods with high nutrient value and those with high enjoyment value.
- Don't restrict or forbid certain types of foods in the home (except if medically necessary such as with a severe food allergy or if financial constraints limit the amount or types of food that can be purchased).
- Don't use food as a reward or punishment (e.g., "You can only have dessert if you eat all your veggies," "We ate too much sugar over the holidays—salads all week!").
- Unlink food/eating from weight (e.g., don't say, "If you keep eating like that, you'll gain weight"). Don't talk about your own diet or restricted eating, especially in the context of trying to change your body size/shape.
- Don't try to control your dancer's portions. Help them connect to and honor their body's hunger and fullness cues and allow them to decide how much they eat.**
- Family meals have been found to protect against dieting, the use of unhealthy weight control practices, and the development of other disordered eating behaviors.[63,64] Try to have meals together as a family more often and create a positive atmosphere during mealtimes that encourages communication and connection with your dancer.

To help dancers develop more balanced and resilient body image:

- Don't comment negatively about your child's body, your own body, or the bodies of others.[32]
- Don't allow others to comment on your child's weight or body. Parents/caregivers may need to request protective practices at medical appointments such as not recommending diets or weight loss and not discussing weight in front of your child (if there are concerns, the doctor can discuss with the parent/caregiver first and then decide how/if to communicate this to your child).
- Don't emphasize body weight/size/shape or appearance as important attributes[32] or reinforce the thin ideal (e.g., by praising or valuing thin bodies and weight loss).

- Help dancers connect with and appreciate non-appearance-based values (e.g., kindness, generosity, resiliency, etc.).
- Foster an appreciation for body diversity. Increase dancers' exposure to bodies of different sizes, shapes, and ability from different cultural, ethnic, and racial backgrounds (e.g., in media and/or in their life).

To support whole dancer health:

- Evaluate your dancer's social media use and its impact on them. Set limits for how much time they spend on social media and when and where they engage with it.[65]
- Help dancers develop an identity separate from dance. Encourage dance/life balance (e.g., by participating and cultivating interest in non-dance activities and socializing with non-dance friends).[40]
- Help dancers nurture a sense of self-worth separate from appearance, achievement, and performance.
- Help dancers develop and practice healthy coping tools to deal with uncomfortable emotions and difficult life circumstances[32] (see Chapters 7 and 9).
- Be a source of support by spending time with your child, having open and compassionate communication, showing them love and attention (especially in difficult times), and accepting them for who they are (and their body as it is).[6,32]

Healthcare Settings

To support dancers in developing good eating habits and prevent dieting:

- Do not recommend restrictive eating practices or diets. Therapeutic diets (i.e., diets that may be indicated for a specific condition, such as a low-FODMAP diet for irritable bowel syndrome) should be recommended with extreme caution and only undertaken with the guidance and close supervision of a dietitian. Even when diet restrictions are medically necessary (e.g., a gluten-free diet for celiac disease), the best practice is to refer to a dietitian to ensure the dancer is meeting their nutrition needs and maintaining a healthy relationship with food.

To support dancers in developing more positive (or neutral) body image:

- If it is necessary to weigh dancers (e.g., to ensure normal growth and development in children/adolescents, during weight restoration in eating disorder recovery), ensure that your weighing practices are eating disorder sensitive and trauma informed. Ask the dancer for permission to be weighed, discuss preferences and recommendations for how it will be done, and if any feedback will be given (e.g., the dancer and/or their treatment team may prefer a blind weight[tt]). Dancers should also consent to and be made aware of who their weight will be shared with (e.g., if the healthcare provider will be sharing the weight with other treatment team members).

- Don't encourage weight loss. On the other hand, if weight gain is needed, it is often helpful for dancers to hear this recommendation from their doctor.
- Don't use judgmental language to discuss weight or weight changes (e.g., "Your weight is good," "You've lost more weight; you must not be following the plan"). Use the terms "biologically appropriate weight" or "estimated minimum weight" instead of "ideal body weight."
- Don't use stigmatizing language such as "skinny," "fat," "overweight," or "obese."

To create a protective environment that supports early intervention:

- Don't dismiss concerns or minimize findings (e.g., "Your labs are fine, so I don't think you have an eating disorder," "Many dancers don't get their periods," "Athletes often have low heart rates").
- Consider the décor and images in your office. Don't hang BMI posters on the wall. Make sure your photos and brochures show diverse body types and individuals of different races, ethnicities, and genders.
- Do not keep diet-promoting magazines in patient areas.

Role Modeling

Dancers learn a lot from what they see their parents, siblings, friends, teachers, and other people they care about and admire do. When dancers observe you eating regular meals and snacks, incorporating a variety of foods, and eating in a way that is nourishing, enjoyable, and flexible, they learn what a healthy relationship with food looks like. When dancers see you honoring your body's needs, hear you speaking kindly about all bodies, and appreciating what your body does for you, they learn what having a neutral and/or positive relationship with your body looks like. When dancers witness you practicing self-compassion, celebrating non-appearance-based attributes, rejecting harmful diet culture messages, and speaking out against diet talk, negative body talk, and body shaming, this shapes their own beliefs and values.

Having healthy role models with food, exercise, and body image can have a profound positive impact on the attitudes and behaviors that dancers develop. My dancer clients often tell me how helpful it is to be around peers and family who have a peaceful relationship with food and their body, and by contrast, how difficult and triggering it can be to be around people who are dieting or speaking negatively about food and bodies.

Modeling healthy habits and a healthy mindset is a powerful way we can support dancers in building these things too. Being a positive role model may not be an easy task if you have been negatively affected by diet and dance culture. You may have your own healing to do, and if so, know that it's never too late and that help is available. Focusing on your own recovery may be one of the most valuable gifts you can give yourself and the dancer(s) in your life.

Main Pointes

- What we communicate to dancers explicitly and implicitly can have a profound and lasting impact.
- We need to carefully consider our language and messaging—especially related to food, eating, weight, and bodies—to ensure we are not exacerbating risk factors for under-fueling, eating disorders, and disordered eating in dancers.
- One of the most beneficial things we can do to protect dancers' health is to prevent them from dieting.
- To help dancers nourish their body optimally and develop a healthy relationship with food: don't label foods as good/bad, use judgmental language to discuss food/eating, or engage in diet talk. Do promote an all foods fit approach and help dancers learn how to tune in to their body's wisdom.
- To decrease the likelihood that dancers will engage in harmful behaviors to change their weight: don't encourage or praise weight loss, don't weigh dancers (in dance settings), and don't engage in or allow weight-based teasing.
- To help dancers develop a more peaceful and accepting relationship with their body: don't engage in or allow negative body talk or body shaming and don't pathologize normal body changes. Do advocate for increased diversity, equity, and inclusion in dance and help dancers practice body image flexibility.
- Self-compassion may be an antidote to multiple risk factors that compromise dancers' physical and mental health.
- Having healthy role models with food, exercise, and body image can have a profound positive impact on the attitudes and behaviors that dancers develop.

Notes

How do you think your own experiences and relationship with food and your body impact your perspective and work with dancers?

Is there any language you have been using (or messages you may have been inadvertently sending) that needs to shift? If so, what can you do and say instead?

Endnotes

* Most dancers with eating disorders/disordered eating will not look "underweight" or have noticeable weight loss.

† These studies use BMI ≥ 25 as an "objective" marker of "overweight." As discussed in Chapter 1, BMI should not be used to determine if an individual's weight is "normal," "healthy," or "over" an arbitrary cut-off. Individuals can have a BMI in the "overweight" range and still be at a weight below where their body functions best.

‡ Weight loss attempts may be somewhat less risky when done with supervision from a qualified professional but still carry risk.

§ i.e., below the weight where their body functions best physically and mentally. A dancer can be underweight even if they don't appear to be at a low weight.

** Under-fueling and eating disorders/disordered eating often lead to suppressed hunger cues. In these situations (depending on the age of the dancer and the type of treatment they are receiving), parents/caregivers may take on more responsibility in what/how much their child eats to help support their recovery.

†† Blind weighing means the dancer doesn't see their weight (e.g., they may get on a scale backwards) and the number is not shared with them.

References

1. Levine MP, Smolak L. The role of protective factors in the prevention of negative body image and disordered eating. *Eat Disord*. 2016;24(1):39–46. doi:10.1080/10640266.2015.1113826

2. National Eating Disorders Collaboration (NEDC). Risk & protective factors. Accessed March 11, 2023. https://nedc.com.au/eating-disorders/eating-disorders-explained/risk-and-protective-factors/

3. Sundgot-Borgen J. Risk and trigger factors for the development of eating disorders in female elite athletes. *Med Sci Sports Exerc*. 1994;26(4):414–419. doi:10.1249/00005768-199404000-00003

4. Dryburgh A, Fortin S. Weighing in on surveillance: Perception of the impact of surveillance on female ballet dancers' health. *Res Dance Educ*. 2010;11(2):95–108. doi:10.1080/14647893.2010.482979

5. Hanson O. First, do no harm: The importance of removing weight stigma from the pediatrician's office. February 26, 2020. Accessed March 11, 2023. https://asdah.org/removing-weight-stigma-from-pediatricians-office/

6. Doria N, Numer M. Dancing in a culture of disordered eating: A feminist poststructural analysis of body and body image among young girls in the world of dance. *PLoS ONE*. 2022;17(1):e0247651. doi:10.1371/journal.pone.0247651

7. Reel JJ, Jamieson KM, SooHoo S, Gill DL. Femininity to the extreme: Body image concerns among college female dancers. *Women Sport Phys Act J*. 2005;14(1):39–51. doi:10.1123/wspaj.14.1.39

8. Heiland TL, Murray DS, Edley PP. Body image of dancers in Los Angeles: The cult of slenderness and media influence among dance students. *Res Dance Educ*. 2008;9(3):257–275. doi:10.1080/14647890802386932

9. Penniment KJ, Egan SJ. Perfectionism and learning experiences in dance class as risk factors for eating disorders in dancers. *Eur Eat Disord Rev*. 2012;20(1):13–22. doi:10.1002/erv.1089

10. Piran N. Eating disorders: A trial of prevention in a high risk school setting. *J Prim Prev*. 1999;20:75–90.

11. Thompson RA, Sherman R. Reflections on athletes and eating disorders. *Psychol Sport Exerc*. 2014;15(6):729–734. doi:10.1016/j.psychsport.2014.06.005

12. O'dea J. School-based interventions to prevent eating problems: First do no harm. *Eat Disord*. 2000;8(2):123–130. doi:10.1080/10640260008251219

13. Keay N, Overseas A, Francis G. Indicators and correlates of low energy availability in male and female dancers. *BMJ Open Sport Exerc Med.* 2020;6(1):e000906. doi:10.1136/bmjsem-2020-000906

14. Hidayah GN, Bariah AHS. Eating attitude, body image, body composition and dieting behaviour among dancers. *Asian J Clin Nutr.* 2011;3(3):92–102. doi:10.3923/ajcn.2011.92.102

15. Gearhart MG, Sugimoto D, Meehan WP, Stracciolini A. Body satisfaction, performance perception, and weight loss behavior in young female dancers. *Med Probl Perform Art.* 2018;33(4):225–230. doi:10.21091/mppa.2018.4033

16. Daly M, Robinson E, Sutin AR. Does knowing hurt? Perceiving oneself as overweight predicts future physical health and well-being. *Psychol Sci.* 2017;28(7):872–881. doi:10.1177/0956797617696311

17. Himmelstein MS, Incollingo Belsky AC, Tomiyama AJ. The weight of stigma: Cortisol reactivity to manipulated weight stigma. *Obesity (Silver Spring).* 2015;23(2):368–374. doi:10.1002/oby.20959

18. Muennig P, Jia H, Lee R, Lubetkin E. I think therefore I am: Perceived ideal weight as a determinant of health. *Am J Public Health.* 2008;98(3):501–506. doi:10.2105/AJPH.2007.114769

19. Ackland TR, Lohman TG, Sundgot-Borgen J, et al. Current status of body composition assessment in sport: Review and position statement on behalf of the ad hoc research working group on body composition health and performance, under the auspices of the I.O.C. Medical Commission. *Sports Med.* 2012;42(3):227–249. doi:10.2165/11597140-000000000-00000

20. Hooper L, Puhl R, Eisenberg ME, Crow S, Neumark-Sztainer D. Weight teasing experienced during adolescence and young adulthood: Cross-sectional and longitudinal associations with disordered eating behaviors in an ethnically/racially and socioeconomically diverse sample. *Int J Eat Disord.* 2021;54(8):1449–1462. doi:10.1002/eat.23534

21. Neumark-Sztainer D, Bauer KW, Friend S, Hannan PJ, Story M, Berge JM. Family weight talk and dieting: How much do they matter for body dissatisfaction and disordered eating behaviors in adolescent girls? *J Adolesc Health.* 2010;47(3):270–276. doi:10.1016/j.jadohealth.2010.02.001

22. Cash TF, Smolak L, eds. *Body Image: A Handbook of Science, Practice, and Prevention.* 2nd ed. The Guilford Press; 2012:490.

23. Eisenberg ME, Neumark-Sztainer D, Story M. Associations of weight-based teasing and emotional well-being among adolescents. *Arch Pediatr Adolesc Med.* 2003;157(8):733–738. doi:10.1001/archpedi.157.8.733

24. Robbeson JG, Kruger HS, Wright HH. Disordered eating behavior, body image, and energy status of female student dancers. *Int J Sport Nutr Exerc Metab.* 2015;25(4):344–352. doi:10.1123/ijsnem.2013-0161

25. Santo André HC, Pinto AJ, Mazzolani BC, et al. "Can a ballerina eat ice cream?": A mixed-method study on eating attitudes and body image in female ballet dancers. *Front Nutr.* 2021;8:665654. doi:10.3389/fnut.2021.665654

26. Arcelus J, García-Dantas A, Sánchez-Martín M, Río-Sanchez C. Influence of perfectionism on variables associated to eating disorders in dancers. *Rev Psicol Deporte.* 2015;24:297–303.

27. Stice E, Marti CN, Durant S. Risk factors for onset of eating disorders: Evidence of multiple risk pathways from an 8-year prospective study. *Behav Res Ther.* 2011;49(10):622–627. doi:10.1016/j.brat.2011.06.009

28. Stice E, Bearman SK. Body-image and eating disturbances prospectively predict increases in depressive symptoms in adolescent girls: A growth curve analysis. *Dev Psychol.* 2001;37(5):597–607. doi:10.1037//0012-1649.37.5.597

29. Černelič-Bizjak M, Jenko-Pražnikar Z. Body dissatisfaction predicts inflammatory status in asymptomatic healthy individuals. *J Health Psychol.* 2018;23(1):25–35. doi:10.1177/1359105316672923

30. Wells KR, Jeacocke NA, Appaneal R, et al. The Australian Institute of Sport (AIS) and National Eating Disorders Collaboration (NEDC) position statement on disordered eating in high performance sport. *Br J Sports Med.* 2020;54(21):1247–1258. doi:10.1136/bjsports-2019-101813

31. Wood-Barcalow N, Tylka T, Judge C. *Positive Body Image Workbook: A Clinical and Self-Improvement Guide.* Cambridge University Press; 2021:372.

32. Loth KA, Neumark-Sztainer D, Croll JK. Informing family approaches to eating disorder prevention: Perspectives of those who have been there. *Int J Eat Disord.* 2009;42(2):146–152. doi:10.1002/eat.20586

33. Webb HJ, Zimmer-Gembeck MJ. The role of friends and peers in adolescent body dissatisfaction: A review and critique of 15 years of research. *J Res Adolesc.* 2014;24(4):564–590. doi:10.1111/jora.12084

34. Shannon A, Mills JS. Correlates, causes, and consequences of fat talk: A review. *Body Image.* 2015;15:158–172. doi:10.1016/j.bodyim.2015.09.003

35. Merriam-Webster. Body-shaming. Accessed March 14, 2023. https://www.merriam-webster.com/dictionary/body-shaming

36. National Association of Anorexia Nervosa and Associated Disorders (ANAD). Body shaming. Accessed March 14, 2023. https://anad.org/get-informed/body-image/body-image-articles/body-shaming/

37. Barnett C. Dancers say it's time to talk about ballet companies that body-shame. November 30, 2020. Accessed March 14, 2023. https://observer.com/2020/11/ballet-companies-body-shaming-kathryn-morgan/

38. Means SP. Ballet alumni described body shaming, bias and intimidation. University of Utah faculty vow continued reform. November 16, 2021. Accessed March 14, 2023. https://www.sltrib.com/artsliving/2021/11/16/ballet-alumni-demand/

39. Klein M, Balsamini D. Ballerina Ashley Bouder says she was body shamed by the NYC Ballet. November 19, 2022. Accessed March 14, 2023. https://nypost.com/2022/11/19/ballerina-ashley-bouder-says-she-was-body-shamed-by-the-nyc-ballet/

40. Kerr G, Berman E, Souza MJD. Disordered eating in women's gymnastics: Perspectives of athletes, coaches, parents, and judges. *J Appl Sport Psychol.* 2006;18(1):28–43. doi:10.1080/10413200500471301

41. Rogol AD, Clark PA, Roemmich JN. Growth and pubertal development in children and adolescents: Effects of diet and physical activity. *Am J Clin Nutr.* 2000;72(2 Suppl):521S–8S. doi:10.1093/ajcn/72.2.521S

42. Wheeler MD. Physical changes of puberty. *Endocrinol Metab Clin North Am.* 1991;20(1):1–14. doi:10.1016/S0889-8529(18)30279-2

43. Mitchell SB, Haase AM, Malina RM, Cumming SP. The role of puberty in the making and breaking of young ballet dancers: Perspectives of dance teachers. *J Adolesc.* 2016;47:81–89. doi:10.1016/j.adolescence.2015.12.007

44. Mainwaring L, Krasnow D. Teaching the dance class: Strategies to enhance skill acquisition, mastery and positive self-image. *J Dance Educ.* 2010;10(1):14–21. doi:10.1080/15290824.2010.10387153

45. Bar RJ, Cassin SE, Dionne MM. The long-term impact of an eating disorder prevention program for professional ballet school students: A 15-year follow-up study. *Eat Disord.* 2017;25(5):375–387. doi:10.1080/10640266.2017.1308731

46. Soulliard ZA, Kauffman AA, Fitterman-Harris HF, Perry JE, Ross MJ. Examining positive body image, sport confidence, flow state, and subjective performance among student athletes and non-athletes. *Body Image.* 2019;28:93–100. doi:10.1016/j.bodyim.2018.12.009

47. Hill ML, Masuda A, Latzman RD. Body image flexibility as a protective factor against disordered eating behavior for women with lower body mass index. *Eat Behav.* 2013;14(3):336–341. doi:10.1016/j.eatbeh.2013.06.003

48. Sandoz EK, Wilson KG, Merwin RM, Kate Kellum K. Assessment of body image flexibility: The body image-acceptance and action questionnaire. *J Contextual Behav Sci.* 2013;2(1–2):39–48. doi:10.1016/j.jcbs.2013.03.002

49. Rogers CB, Webb JB, Jafari N. A systematic review of the roles of body image flexibility as correlate, moderator, mediator, and in intervention science (2011–2018). *Body Image.* 2018;27:43–60. doi:10.1016/j.bodyim.2018.08.003

50. Albertson ER, Neff KD, Dill-Shackleford KE. Self-compassion and body dissatisfaction in women: A randomized controlled trial of a brief meditation intervention. *Mindfulness.* 2015;6(3):444–454. doi:10.1007/s12671-014-0277-3

51. Neff KD. Self-compassion, self-esteem, and well-being. *Soc Personal Psychol Compass.* 2011;5(1):1–12. doi:10.1111/j.1751-9004.2010.00330.x

52. Sirois FM, Kitner R, Hirsch JK. Self-compassion, affect, and health-promoting behaviors. *Health Psychol.* 2015;34(6):661–669. doi:10.1037/hea0000158

53. Neff K. Why self-compassion is healthier than self-esteem. Accessed March 15, 2023. https://self-compassion.org/why-self-compassion-is-healthier-than-self-esteem/

54. Radell SA, Mandradjieff MP, Adame DD, Cole SP. Impact of mirrors on body image of beginning modern and ballet students. *J Dance Med Sci.* 2020;24(3):126–134. doi:10.12678/1089-313X.24.3.126

55. Dantas AG, Alonso DA, Sánchez-Miguel PA, Del Río Sánchez C. Factors dancers associate with their body dissatisfaction. *Body Image.* 2018;25:40–47. doi:10.1016/j.bodyim.2018.02.003

56. Radell SA, IADMS Dance Educators' Committee. Mirrors in the dance class: Help or hindrance. Published online 2019. Accessed March 16, 2023. https://iadms.org/media/5781/iadms-resource-paper-mirrors-in-the-dance-class.pdf

57. Hornthal E. The dance studio mirror: Reflection vs. reflecting. August 28, 2018. Accessed March 16, 2023. https://www.danceinforma.com/2018/08/28/the-dance-studio-mirror-reflection-vs-reflecting/

58. Nicholls C. Is it time to rethink how we use mirrors in dance? May 5, 2021. Accessed March 16, 2023. https://www.dancemagazine.com/mirrors-in-dance-classes/

59. Biesecker AC, Martz DM. Impact of coaching style on vulnerability for eating disorders: An analog study. *Eat Disord.* 1999;7(3):235–244. doi:10.1080/10640269908249289

60. Currie A. Sport and eating disorders – Understanding and managing the risks. *Asian J Sports Med.* 2010;1(2):63–68. doi:10.5812/asjsm.34864

61. Seibert B. Black in ballet: Coming together after trying to 'blend into the corps.' *The New York Times.* August 17, 2021. Accessed July 24, 2022. https://www.nytimes.com/2021/08/17/arts/dance/misty-copeland-little-island.html.

62. Swarting L. How to develop a safe and successful dance partnership. January 12, 2022. Accessed March 16, 2023. https://pointemagazine.com/how-to-develop-a-safe-and-successful-dance-partnership/

63. Haines J, Gillman MW, Rifas-Shiman S, Field AE, Austin SB. Family dinner and disordered eating behaviors in a large cohort of adolescents. *Eat Disord.* 2010;18(1):10–24. doi:10.1080/10640260903439516

64. Loth K, Wall M, Choi C-W, et al. Family meals and disordered eating in adolescents: Are the benefits the same for everyone? *Int J Eat Disord.* 2015;48(1):100–110. doi:10.1002/eat.22339

65. The Full Bloom Project. *The ABCs of body-positive parenting.* 2019.

Act III
Nourishing the Whole Dancer

6 Gentle Nutrition for Dancers

Food is fuel AND something to enjoy, not either/or.
~female ballet dancer

Why Gentle Nutrition?

I've borrowed the term "gentle nutrition" from the authors of *Intuitive Eating*[1] to highlight the importance of dancers learning how to fuel their bodies in a way that is gentle rather than harsh, rigid, or punishing. Taking this gentle approach helps nourish the whole dancer and doesn't sacrifice mental health and well-being for the sake of meeting nutrition goals. Gentle nutrition is compassionate and embraces the fact that there is no such thing as perfect eating.

Optimal fueling for dancers means their diet provides necessary nutrients and supports performance and recovery; is adaptable, flexible, and enjoyable; and is free of restrictive eating practices.[2] As shown in Figure 6.1, honoring the interconnectedness between what dancers eat, their relationship with food, and their health and performance is critical. This chapter explores fundamental aspects of nutrition for dancers beginning with a discussion of what, when, and how much to eat. These recommendations are meant to be gentle guidelines (not rules) that can be adapted to best meet each dancer's individual needs, preferences, and circumstances.

What to Eat: Macronutrients

Almost everything we eat is made up of one or more of the macronutrients—carbohydrates, protein, and fat. We need macronutrients in relatively large amounts (hence the name), and we need all three for our body to function optimally.

Carbohydrates

Carbohydrates (aka carbs) are unfairly villainized in diet culture, which contributes to some dancers under-consuming this essential nutrient.

DOI: 10.4324/9781003366171-9

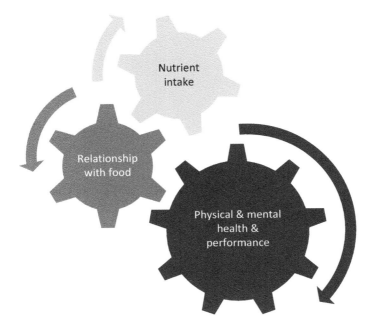

Figure 6.1 Optimal Fueling for Dancers.

The main function of carbohydrates is to provide energy. Carbohydrates are the preferred fuel for most of the body's functions and are especially important for the brain and muscles—two things that dancers use a lot! Eating enough carbohydrates throughout the day is essential to help dancers maintain high levels of energy and focus.

Other roles of carbohydrates include:

• Maintaining blood sugar levels.
• Providing fiber, which helps keep the digestive tract healthy and working smoothly.
• Sparing protein. Eating enough carbohydrates prevents protein from being used as an energy source (and consequently prevents muscle from being broken down to provide protein for this purpose).[3] The protein-sparing function of carbohydrates keeps protein available to perform all its critical jobs in the body.

The Truth about Carbs

Regardless of the source—whether from quinoa or gummy bears—carbohydrates are broken down into the same thing (i.e., glucose), which the body uses as fuel or stores as glycogen for later use. I am not saying that whole grains and candy are nutritionally equivalent or interchangeable. However, it's helpful to understand how your body digests and uses carbohydrates. The body is capable of using all foods (with macronutrients) as fuel, including sugar. In fact, because simple sugars are rapidly digested, they can be useful in sports nutrition.

Carb TIP: Carbohydrates should make up more than half of a dancer's diet, which means that of the three macronutrients, dancers need the most carbohydrates. I don't recommend "counting macros," but am sharing this information to highlight how important carbohydrates are for dancers and why low-carb diets are not appropriate.

Table 6.1 lists sources of carbohydrates (as well as protein and fat). This list is not all-inclusive—there are many other foods that provide macronutrients. Some foods contain more than one kind of macronutrient. For example, beans/lentils provide both carbohydrates and protein, and nuts provide protein and fat. Milk and yogurt contain carbohydrates and protein, and depending on type, may also be a source of fat.

Non-starchy vegetables (like spinach, tomatoes, cauliflower, etc.) don't provide much carbohydrate per serving. There are lots of good reasons to eat vegetables including for the fiber, vitamins, minerals, and phytochemicals they offer, but non-starchy vegetables shouldn't be the main source of carbohydrates for dancers. Dancers need to include a variety of other foods from the carbohydrate group to ensure they consume enough of this important nutrient.

Table 6.1 Macronutrient Sources

Carbohydrate	Protein	Fat
Grains: rice, barley, bulgur, oats, pasta, cereal, bread, etc.	Meat	Oil (e.g., olive, canola)
Quinoa, buckwheat	Poultry (e.g., chicken, turkey)	Butter
Starchy vegetables: corn, peas, potatoes, plantains	Fish and seafood	Fatty fish (e.g., salmon, sardines)
Non-starchy vegetables[a]	Eggs	Salad dressing
Beans/lentils	Beans/lentils	Hummus
Fruit	Nuts and seeds	Nuts and seeds
Milk and yogurt	Dairy (milk, cheese, yogurt)	Coconut
Sugar and sweeteners (e.g., honey, maple syrup)	Tofu and other soy foods	Olives
Desserts and sweets	Seitan	Avocado

[a]Non-starchy vegetables do not provide much carbohydrate per serving.

Protein

Most dancers know protein is important for their muscles. One of the main functions of protein is muscle building and repair. Consuming enough protein is essential to help dancers maintain and improve strength and is critical for recovery from training.

Protein is also needed for:

- Growth and repair of tissues. The body's cells and tissues are constantly being replaced and these processes require protein. In addition to this role in body maintenance, protein is also needed for healing—whether it's a small blister or a more serious injury.
- Healthy ligaments, tendons, cartilage, bones, and skin.
- Making enzymes, which are necessary for countless body functions including breaking down the food we eat to get energy.
- A healthy immune system (e.g., antibodies are proteins that help protect us from infection and illness).
- Making some hormones (e.g., thyroid hormones, insulin).[3]

Protein TIP: Dancers should try to include protein in each meal and snack. Distributing protein consumption evenly throughout the day (vs. eating very little at some meals and then having a large amount at once) enhances muscle building and repair.[4]

Fat

Though some dancers shun fat (often related to the mistaken belief that eating fat will cause weight gain), fear of this nutrient seems to be decreasing, perhaps due to the recent popularity of high-fat diets (e.g., "keto") or diet culture's embrace of avocado and nuts. Like the other two macronutrients, fat is essential for dancers. It provides an additional source of energy for the body and is needed to help absorb fat-soluble nutrients (i.e., vitamins A, D, E, K). Fat often makes food taste better and improves satiety and satisfaction. Enjoying what we eat is an important part of healthy eating!

Other key roles of fat in the body include:

- Brain and nerve functioning
- Hormone production (e.g., estrogen, testosterone)
- Protecting organs and bones (by serving as a shock absorber)
- Temperature regulation

Fat TIP: Omega-3 fatty acids help reduce inflammation. Sources include fatty fish (e.g., salmon, tuna, sardines), walnuts, ground flaxseed, flaxseed oil, chia seeds, and hemp seeds.

What to Eat: Micronutrients

Although micronutrients (aka vitamins and minerals) are needed in much smaller amounts than macronutrients, they are essential for health and have powerful roles in the body. Vitamins and minerals are critical for growth and development, for maintaining normal body functions, and for disease prevention. For example, consuming enough iron can help prevent anemia and adequate calcium intake helps prevent osteoporosis. This section will focus on a few key micronutrients for dancers. Calcium, vitamin D, and iron often require extra attention to ensure needs are met.[5-7] Recommended amounts for these three micronutrients are provided in the chapter endnotes.

Calcium

Calcium is perhaps best known for its critical role in building and maintaining strong bones. It is also necessary for healthy teeth, proper muscle functioning, and nerve transmission.[8] Dairy is one of the best sources of calcium and also provides other nutrients (e.g., vitamin D, phosphorus, potassium, magnesium, and protein) that are important for bone health.[9] Not surprisingly, higher dairy intake is associated with better bone density in dancers.[10] Dancers who avoid or limit dairy products and those who are under-fueling are at risk for inadequate calcium consumption.[11]

Dancers require a higher intake of calcium during their critical bone-building years.[†] To meet their calcium needs, dancers should aim for 3–4 daily servings of dairy (milk, cheese, yogurt) or a non-dairy calcium equivalent. For example, each of these choices has a similar amount of calcium as one cup of dairy milk[12]:

- Cup of calcium-fortified plant milk
- Cup of calcium-fortified orange juice
- Fist-sized portion of cooked kale or collard greens
- Palm- to hand-sized portion of tofu (calcium-set)
- Palm-sized portion of canned sardines (with bones)

Although the above foods/beverages are good sources of calcium, some are lacking protein and/or vitamin D (see Nourishing Tips for Dancers for recommendations on dairy alternatives).

Vitamin D

Vitamin D is calcium's partner in bone health. It helps us absorb calcium and maintains blood levels of calcium and phosphorus, which are necessary functions for building and maintaining healthy bones.[13] Vitamin D is also important for our immune system and plays a role in muscle strength and function and reducing inflammation.[14]

Vitamin D is known as the "sunshine vitamin" because it can be made when skin is exposed to sunlight. Because sun exposure is a major source of vitamin D, factors that affect dancers' exposure to or absorption of the ultraviolet rays of the sun (e.g., training indoors, living above the southern border of Tennessee,‡ darker skin,§ wearing sunscreen) also impact vitamin D levels.[11,15] Food sources of vitamin D include[12,15]:

- Fortified foods (e.g., dairy, plant milk, cereal)
- Fatty fish (e.g., salmon, sardines, tuna)
- Egg yolks
- UV- or sun-exposed mushrooms

Vitamin D is fat-soluble, so consuming it with fat helps absorption. However, meeting requirements via diet alone is difficult.

Dancers often require vitamin D supplementation to meet their needs, especially during the winter months when insufficiency/deficiency is more likely.[16] It's useful for dancers to have their vitamin D levels checked to determine if a supplement is needed, and if so, what dosage is appropriate. There is current debate over the requirements for vitamin D with varying amounts suggested by different organizations.**,[17]

Magnesium

Magnesium is another important nutrient for bone health and muscle function.[14] Magnesium also has roles in nerve transmission, neuromuscular coordination, and blood sugar control and is necessary for the body processes that turn the food we eat into energy.[18,19] There are a variety of good food sources of magnesium including[12]:

- Nuts (e.g., almonds, cashews, peanuts)
- Seeds (e.g., chia, pumpkin, hemp)
- Beans
- Whole grains (e.g., brown rice, oats, whole grain pasta)
- Potatoes
- Spinach
- Dark chocolate

Unfortunately, dancers have been found to have low intakes of this micronutrient,[5] which may be related to under-fueling.

Spotlight on Bone Health

As discussed in Chapter 2, late childhood through adolescence is a critical time for bone building[20] with 90% of peak bone mass acquired by age 18–20.[21] The peak bone mass (i.e., the maximum bone density and strength)[21] that a dancer attains will impact skeletal health throughout their life.[22] Beginning in our thirties, we are no longer able to increase total bone mass.[20] We continue remodeling our bones—breaking down old bone and replacing it with new bone—but the breakdown starts to happen faster than the building,[23] and the goal shifts from optimizing nutrition for bone building to optimizing nutrition to minimize bone loss.

Regardless of the phase of life dancers are in, eating enough of the nutrients that support bone health is key. In addition to calcium, vitamin D, and magnesium, other important micronutrients for bone health include phosphorus[††] (found in dairy, meat/poultry, fish, nuts, beans/lentils), potassium (found in fruit, vegetables, dairy, beans/lentils), vitamin C (see below for sources), and vitamin K (found in green leafy vegetables like collard greens, spinach, kale, and broccoli). Consuming adequate energy (aka calories) and macronutrients is also essential for building and maintaining strong, healthy bones.

Iron

Iron is a key component of the oxygen-carrying proteins hemoglobin (in red blood cells) and myoglobin (in muscle). Hemoglobin carries oxygen from the lungs to the rest of the body and myoglobin carries and stores oxygen for use by the muscles.[3] Iron also has roles in energy metabolism (i.e., getting energy from the food we eat) and cognitive function.[18]

Iron deficiency occurs on a spectrum of severity from depleted iron stores to iron deficiency anemia,[††,24] and can have a significant negative impact on a dancer's health and performance.[11] Symptoms of iron deficiency (which are usually more pronounced with anemia)[25] include low energy/fatigue, weakness, decreased endurance, dizziness, shortness of breath during exercise, and cold hands and feet.[25-27] Studies have found that iron deficiency is common in female dancers.[5,28] Research on male dancers is lacking; however, based on studies in athletes, iron deficiency occurs frequently in male athletes as well.[29,30]

Multiple factors contribute to the elevated risk of iron deficiency in dancers. Inadequate iron intake is a major cause of deficiency, and under-fueling increases the likelihood of low iron consumption.[11] Dancers with high training loads are at greater risk for deficiency because iron is lost in sweat, and exercise increases the breakdown of red blood cells.[25,27] Iron is also lost in blood; therefore, menstruating dancers are at greater risk for deficiency, especially those with heavy bleeding.[27] Iron requirements for females of reproductive age are higher than for males and post-menopausal females because of menstrual blood loss.[§§]

Good sources of iron include[12]:

- Red meat
- Turkey/chicken

- Shellfish (e.g., oysters, mussels)
- Beans/lentils
- Nuts/seeds (e.g., cashews, pumpkin seeds)
- Spinach
- Fortified foods (e.g., cereal)

Iron in food comes in two forms—heme (in meat, poultry, fish) and non-heme (in plant sources and fortified foods). Non-heme iron is not as well absorbed as heme iron. Consequently, vegan/vegetarian dancers may need up to 1.8 times more iron than those who eat meat.[31] It may take some planning to meet these higher iron requirements.[27] As one example, consuming two fist-sized portions of iron-fortified cereal, one cup of soy milk, a fist-sized portion each of cooked spinach and lentils, and a handful of pumpkin seeds would provide the daily recommended amount of iron for a 20-year-old, vegetarian dancer who menstruates.[12,31]

Substances present in coffee, tea, whole grains, and legumes impair iron absorption.[3] On the other hand, vitamin C greatly enhances the absorption of iron from non-heme sources. Dancers who are trying to improve their iron stores benefit from avoiding excessive intake of coffee and tea and separating consumption of these beverages from meals. Pairing iron-rich foods with a good source of vitamin C is another helpful strategy to improve absorption (e.g., adding strawberries to iron-fortified cereal).

Some dancers may need an iron supplement to correct deficiency, especially if they have anemia.[27] However, it is not recommended to supplement without first consulting with a doctor or healthcare professional. Calcium may interfere with iron absorption, so dancers taking both types of supplements should take them at different times of the day.[31] Ideally, dancers would have their iron status regularly assessed with a blood test[32] that checks not just for anemia but also for earlier signs of deficiency such as reduced iron stores (i.e., serum ferritin level).[31] Dancers with iron deficiency should have ongoing monitoring to evaluate the effectiveness of dietary interventions and/or supplementation.

Vitamin C

Vitamin C is needed to make collagen, which is an essential component of bones, tendons, ligaments, and other connective tissues. It also has important roles in wound and injury healing and immune function and is a powerful antioxidant. Prolonged and/or intense exercise increases the production of compounds called free radicals, which can cause damage in the body if they are not counteracted.[3] Antioxidants, such as vitamin C, are part of the body's defense system that stops the negative effects of free radicals.

Athletes (including dancers) likely have somewhat higher requirements for vitamin C than less active individuals,[33] but needs can be easily met with food, especially with a diet plentiful in fruit and vegetables. For example, a dancer can get the recommended daily amount of vitamin C by eating a kiwi, a fist-sized portion of strawberries, and a tennis ball-sized portion of cooked broccoli. Other excellent sources of vitamin C include[12]:

- Oranges
- Grapefruit
- Pineapple
- Green and red peppers
- Brussels sprouts

Dancers don't need (and shouldn't take) high-dose vitamin C supplements, which have been shown to impair adaptation to training.[34]

Food vs. Supplements

It's preferable for dancers to get their micronutrients by eating a balanced and varied diet that provides enough energy. This food first approach provides vitamins and minerals plus the health benefits of other components in food (e.g., macronutrients, fiber, phytochemicals) that are not present in supplements or may not offer the same advantages when they come in supplement form. Getting nutrients from food also prevents the negative consequences that may result from taking unnecessary supplements.

More is not better when it comes to vitamins and minerals. Unfortunately, many supplements (especially mega-dose varieties) have excessive amounts of vitamins and/or minerals and may contain other substances that can be risky for dancers. By contrast, it is unlikely that harmful levels of vitamins and minerals will be consumed from food alone. In addition, some vitamin, mineral, and herbal supplements can interact with medications or other supplements and cause undesirable or potentially dangerous side effects.

Dietary supplements are not well regulated in the U.S. The Food and Drug Administration (FDA) does not test or approve supplements for safety, purity, or effectiveness, nor do they ensure accurate or truthful labeling before supplements are sold.[35] Lack of oversight of the supplement industry contributes to a plethora of misleading claims about the benefits of supplements as well as products on the market that contain unlisted, adulterated, and prohibited ingredients, and/or amounts far greater or less than indicated on the label.[36]

Supplements may be needed if dancers are not able to meet their micronutrient requirements with diet alone or to correct a deficiency (e.g., vitamin D and iron as discussed above or to meet higher needs of pregnancy). Dancers with conditions that affect absorption of nutrients (e.g., celiac disease, Crohn's disease) and those with limited or restricted diets (e.g., dancers who are selective eaters, allergic to multiple foods, vegan, or under-fueling) may require a multivitamin and mineral supplement and/or other individual micronutrient supplements. For example, dancers following a vegan diet need to get vitamin B12 either in a supplement or fortified foods. Dancers should get guidance from their doctor or dietitian before taking any supplements.

When purchasing supplements, choose products that have been certified by a third-party organization (e.g., U.S. Pharmacopeia [USP], NSF Certified for Sport®), which provide some assurances regarding the supplement's quality and safety.

Hydration

Hydration status affects energy levels, recovery from training, and injury risk, and being even slightly underhydrated can impair performance.[32,33,37] Signs and symptoms of hypohydration include thirst, flushed skin, fatigue, headache, lightheadedness/dizziness, stomach (and possibly muscle[***]) cramps, and nausea.[37] Dehydration can also worsen cognitive function[38] and impact concentration[39] and memory,[40] making it harder to pick up and execute choreography. Hydration is clearly an important factor for dancers' health and performance.

Dancers shouldn't wait until they feel thirsty to drink.[32] Instead, it's beneficial to build a hydration routine that includes drinking ample amounts of fluid before/after dance and with meals/snacks, as well as sipping fluids frequently during classes and rehearsals.[32] The goal is for dancers to start their dance day well hydrated, maintain hydration during dance, and replace fluid and electrolyte losses post-dance (but not consume excessive fluid which can be dangerous).[37] To support these hydration goals, it's better for dancers to drink fluids regularly throughout the day rather than go long periods with minimal intake followed by having large volumes of fluid at one time.

Fluid needs vary substantially based on factors such as age, sex, body size, medical conditions, activity amount and intensity, sweat rate, and environment. The Institute of Medicine established the following Adequate Intake (AI) levels for daily water[41]:

- Age 9–13: Boys: 2.4 L (≈10 cups), Girls: 2.1 L (≈9 cups)
- Age 14–18: Boys: 3.3 L (≈14 cups), Girls: 2.3 L (≈9.5 cups)
- Age 19+: Men: 3.7 L (≈15.5 cups), Women: 2.7 L (≈11.5 cups)

Dancers require more than this as these estimates are not specific for athletes and therefore do not account for fluid losses of training and performing (higher amounts are also needed during pregnancy and lactation).[41] If you are thinking, "that's a lot of water!," keep in mind that these recommendations are for total water intake, which includes fluid from all food and beverages. Food supplies about 20% of the water we need[41]—another good reason not to skip meals and snacks.

Everything dancers eat and drink that contains water (coffee, tea, juice, milk, smoothies, soup, fruit, vegetables, etc.) helps meet their fluid needs. Water is usually the best beverage choice for dancers; however, there are some situations in which sports drinks (e.g., Gatorade, Powerade) may be preferable. For example, sports drinks that contain carbohydrates can be use-ful for dancers with high energy needs or those who are dancing for extended periods without a long enough break to consume adequate fuel via food. Sports drinks also provide electrolytes which can help replace losses from profuse sweating (e.g., when training or performing in hot/humid conditions or for dancers who sweat a lot).

Dancers should be cautious with caffeinated beverages because excessive[†††] consumption can cause jitteriness, increase anxiety, and interfere with sleep. Energy drinks, which are often classified as dietary supplements, are not well regulated in the U.S.[42] and are not recommended for dancers. These bever-ages typically contain caffeine (sometimes at high levels) and/or other stimu-lants and may include potentially harmful ingredients (or combinations of ingredients).[42,43] According to the American Academy of Pediatrics, due to the potential health risks, energy drinks should never be consumed by chil-dren or adolescents.[44]

Hydration TIP: Urine color provides some insight into hydration status. Pale yellow urine (e.g., color of lemonade) is a sign of adequate fluid intake, whereas darker urine (e.g., color of apple juice) is an indicator of hypohy-dration.[33] Certain vitamin supplements (e.g., B vitamins) change the color of urine[33] making the "pee-test" less useful. The frequency and volume of urine also reflect hydration status, and when either is reduced, this may indicate the need for additional fluid intake.

Meal Planning for Dancers

Now that you know which nutrients are important for dancers, let's discuss what fueling might look like in terms of meals and snacks. I usually use the template shown in Figure 6.2 when doing meal planning for dancers. By focusing on including these four food groups (i.e., starch/grain, protein and/ or dairy, fruit and/or vegetables, and fat) at three meals a day, dancers will be a good way toward meeting their nutritional needs. The beauty of this tem-plate is that it works with all types of foods, preferences, and cuisines, and in most situations. It also provides flexibility so that dancers can nourish their body well whether they are at home, at school, in the studio, at a restaurant, on tour, or on vacation.

Though the arrows for each of the food groups are the same size, this is not meant as a recommendation to make the portions of each group the same. Dancers need more carbohydrates than protein or fat, so making starches/grains (e.g., rice, pasta, quinoa, bread, cereal, potatoes) the founda-tion of meals is optimal. Fruit and (some) dairy products also provide car-bohydrates, but generally should proportionally make up a smaller part of meals than starches/grains. In addition to three meals a day with these four components, most dancers need two to three daily snacks (though some-times more or less) to meet their nutrient requirements and be well fueled.

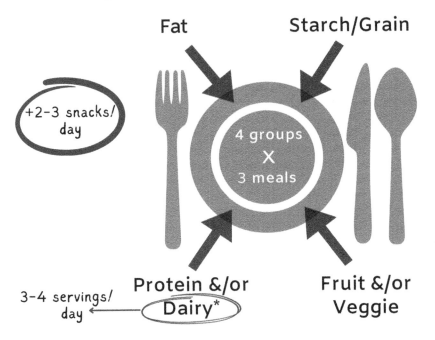

Figure 6.2 Meal Planning Template for Dancers.

Created by the author (image credit © nikiteev, © sparklestroke, and © maddie-red-images via Canva.com). *Dairy or calcium equivalent.

For most snacks, I recommend including a good source of carbohydrate (e.g., starch, grain, fruit) plus a protein and/or dairy food (other food groups can be included as well). This carbohydrate plus protein combination provides sustained energy and tends to be most satisfying (see the Meal Timing section for additional snack guidelines). Portion sizes for meals and snacks will vary based on each dancer's individual needs.

Remember we are striving for a *gentle* approach to nutrition. Therefore, these recommendations should be viewed as guidelines rather than rules. Dancers won't develop a sudden nutrient deficiency if they don't follow this template perfectly at every meal and snack. It is the food choices that dancers make most of the time and how and what they eat consistently over time that will have the greatest impact on their health and performance.

Nourishing Tips for Dancers

To help dancers put together nourishing meals and snacks that honor their needs as individuals and in different situations, consider the following:

- Whole grains typically provide more fiber and are more nutrient dense than refined grains. Most dancers benefit from aiming to make at least half of their grain choices whole (unless they have a digestive condition or other issue that makes refined grains preferable more/most of the time).

- Refined (aka "white") grains lose some nutrients in processing; however, many of these products are enriched and/or fortified with added vitamins and minerals. Refined grains are easier to digest and provide a quicker source of fuel, which is helpful close to or during activity. Refined grains may also be a food preference or cultural staple (e.g., white rice) that can absolutely fit into a healthy diet.
- Including a variety of foods from each of the food groups helps dancers meet their nutrient needs and enhances health. For example, by eating fruits and vegetables of all colors, dancers get the health benefits of consuming diverse phytochemicals as well as varying types and amounts of vitamins and minerals.
- Calcium is critical. Dancers should include 3–4 daily servings of dairy (or calcium equivalent) in meals and/or snacks to meet their needs. For dancers who do not consume dairy, it's helpful to choose substitutes that are fortified with calcium and vitamin D and contain similar amounts of protein as dairy (e.g., soy milk, pea milk, or oat/nut milks with added protein).
- Busy schedules make planning ahead necessary. Dancers will be much more likely to be well fueled if they have easy-to-eat meals and snacks on hand.
- Pleasure is a part of healthy eating. Encourage dancers to eat foods they enjoy and that are satisfying.
- There is no such thing as "perfect" eating. All foods can fit.

Meal Ideas for Dancers

A few examples of easy meals that incorporate all four food categories are listed below. They are suggested as breakfast, lunch, and dinner, but any of the choices can be eaten at any time. However, for meals that occur during the dance day, nutrient-dense, lower-volume options (e.g., sandwich instead of a salad) work best for most dancers. The meals can easily be made gluten-free (e.g., by replacing the grain with a gluten-free choice), and/or vegan/vegetarian (e.g., by replacing meat with tofu, tempeh, or seitan), and can be adapted to incorporate cultural foods and practices.

Breakfast

- Oatmeal made with milk (or cereal with milk) topped with banana and nuts
- Veggie egg scramble served in a wrap with cheese and/or avocado plus a side of fruit
- Smoothie made with milk, fruit, nut butter, and protein powder (optional), topped with granola
- Waffles topped with Greek yogurt or nut butter, fruit, and syrup/honey drizzle

Lunch

- Peanut butter and sliced apple sandwich with a side of yogurt and berries
- Turkey, cheese, baby spinach, tomato, and avocado sandwich with a side of pretzels and fruit
- Pasta salad made with chicken, feta cheese, tomatoes, cucumbers, olives and dressed with oil and lemon
- Snack box style: crackers, cheese, hard-boiled egg, baby carrots, hummus, and grapes

Dinner

- Stir fry with protein of choice (chicken, shrimp, tofu, etc.), broccoli, cabbage, and carrots cooked with sesame oil and served with rice
- Burger (beef, turkey, veggie, etc.) with cheese on a bun plus a side salad with dressing
- Salmon, roasted sweet potatoes, and grilled asparagus topped with pesto
- Burrito bowl with rice, beans, protein of choice (chicken, beef, seitan, etc.), cheese, lettuce, tomatoes, peppers, onions, and guacamole

Snack Ideas for Dancers

Table 6.2 lists some snack options for dancers that contain carbohydrates and protein (this is not an exhaustive list—there are many other choices!). In addition, it's not necessary to eat "snack foods" for snacks. Some dancers may prefer to have smaller portions of the foods they eat at meals (e.g., chicken and rice) instead.

When to Eat: Meal Timing for Dancers

It's not just *what* dancers eat, but also *when* they eat that's important. I often work with dancers who skip breakfast because they wake up late or aren't hungry, eat a small lunch because they have limited time and don't want to feel full while dancing, and then they are "starving" at night and consume the majority of their nutrients after their dance day is over. Unfortunately, even if dancers are getting enough total nutrition (though that's difficult to do with a pattern like described), being in an under-fueled state at times during the day can have negative consequences for their health and performance (see Within-Day Energy Deficiency section in Chapter 2).

Getting balanced, consistent, and sufficient nutrition throughout the day is the foundation of optimal fueling for dancers. I typically recommend that dancers try to eat within one hour of waking because they've been fasting overnight and need to get fuel into their system to power the first part of their day. After this, dancers should aim to have a meal or snack about every 3–4 hours,[4,32] though some dancers find it easier to meet their needs if they eat more frequently.

Table 6.2 Sustaining Snacks for Dancers

Mix and Match Options—Select One or More Items[a] from the Carb and Protein Groups		
Carbohydrate	*+ Protein*	*Examples*
Cereal Bread Crackers Pretzels Granola/granola bar Fruit (fresh, dried)	Cheese Yogurt Milk (dairy, soy, pea) Nuts/seeds Nut butter Hard-boiled egg Meat/fish (e.g., jerky, turkey/chicken slices, canned or pouched tuna/salmon)	Crackers + cheese Pretzels + turkey jerky Cereal + milk Toast + almond butter Banana + peanut butter Apple + parmesan crisps Trail mix (nuts, dried fruit, cereal) Granola + yogurt Granola bar + glass of milk Pita chips + hard-boiled egg Fruit + turkey and cheese roll-up Crackers + tuna salad
Combination Snacks[a]		
Energy bars that contain carbs and protein (e.g., Clif, GoMacro, RX, Kind, Luna, etc.)[b] Roasted chickpeas Edamame Chocolate milk Smoothie (made with fruit + milk, yogurt, and/or protein powder)		

[a]Portion sizes vary based on needs.
[b]Bars differ widely in nutrition content, taste, texture, and price. The best bar for a dancer is the one that best suits their needs and preferences.

By paying attention to nutrient timing around and during dance (and other physical activity), dancers can level up their nutrition plan to increase energy and focus, improve recovery, and help prevent injury. As mentioned above, some dancers under-fuel because of lack of hunger and/or discomfort with eating close to dance. In many cases, when dancers get into the habit of eating consistently, hunger cues improve. In addition, the digestive system can be trained to better absorb and tolerate fuel, making it more comfortable to consume food/beverages before and during activity.[45]

Dancers' schedules as well as the frequency, volume, and intensity of training and performing differ substantially based on factors such as genre, level, type of dance environment (e.g., recreational setting, competition studio, pre-professional program, college program, company) and the time in the season (e.g., performance season vs. layoff period). Using the framework presented here, dancers can adapt fueling strategies to best meet their individual and changing needs. Following the pre-, during, and post-dance recommendations is especially important for dancers who are training and/or performing multiple hours a day, several days a week (though the approach should remain gentle and flexible). Dancers who take a single class a few times a week or who are on a break may not need as careful attention to meeting these nutrient timing goals. Though not listed below, adequate hydration is also vital in each period.

Fueling before Dance

3–4 hours before: A balanced meal that includes carbohydrates, protein, and some fat is generally well tolerated. If there is less time between eating and dance, dancers usually benefit from smaller portions and easier-to-digest options as described below.

2 hours before: As dancers get closer to activity, fat and fiber should be reduced because they slow down digestion and may cause abdominal discomfort. For example, 3–4 hours before dance, a turkey, cheese, vegetable, and avocado sandwich on whole grain bread with a couple of side items could be a nourishing meal. Two hours before dance, it might feel better to remove the vegetables and avocado, use sourdough bread, and skip the sides or replace them with juice. It's important to note that there is a tremendous amount of variability in what will work best for a dancer—some may feel fine eating a fuller meal two hours before dance.

15–60 minutes before: If a dancer eats 3–4 hours before dance, they will need an additional snack to top off their energy stores before class, rehearsal, or a performance. Depending on individual needs, prior intake, and the volume and intensity of dancing, this might be two hours before and/or within an hour of activity.[23] Fifteen minutes to one hour before, the snack should contain mostly carbohydrates and be quickly digested (e.g., fresh or dried fruit, applesauce, pretzels, sports drink).

Staying Well Fueled during Dance

Dancers need extra fuel during back-to-back classes, long rehearsals or performance days, or any time they are dancing for several hours without sufficient breaks to eat.[11] To keep energy levels up and focus sharp, dancers can take bites of carbohydrate foods that are quickly digested and absorbed (e.g., applesauce, clementine segments, dried fruit, gummy candy, pretzels) or sip on a sports drink. The amount of fuel needed during dance will depend on the intensity and duration of dancing.

Re-fueling after Dance

0–60 minutes after: As soon as possible after dance (within the first hour), dancers should have a snack or meal that contains easy-to-digest carbohydrates plus protein (e.g., low-fat chocolate milk, fruit smoothie made with milk and/ or protein powder, juice and a protein bar).[4,46,47] This is an important period for recovery during which carbohydrates are needed to replenish the fuel (i.e., glycogen) used while dancing and protein is needed for muscle repair. Prioritizing recovery nutrition is always important, but rapid re-fueling is even more vital if a dancer will be dancing again in less than 8 hours[47] (e.g., on a two-show day or a day with both rehearsals and a performance).

2–4 hours after: The next few hours after dancing remain critical for the recovery process as a dancer's body continues to restore and repair. After the initial recovery meal or snack, dancers need to eat again a few hours later. Including antioxidant-rich foods (e.g., fruits and vegetables) and anti-inflammatory omega-3 fatty acids (found in salmon, tuna, flaxseed oil, etc.) in this meal/snack can aid in recovery.[48] The more intense a dancer's schedule is, the more critical optimizing recovery is.

Special Considerations for Auditions and Performances

Nerves can impact appetite and hunger cues and cause digestive symptoms (e.g., nausea, early satiety, diarrhea) that make it more challenging to fuel adequately. Even if dancers don't feel like eating, their body needs fuel to perform at their best. In these situations, liquid meals like smoothies usually work well. Incorporating coping strategies for stress and anxiety (e.g., breathing or grounding exercises, meditation) into a pre-performance or pre-audition routine can also make it easier to eat. Dancers should use rehearsals to practice their fueling plan. It's best not to try new foods or beverages on the day of a performance or audition.

How Much to Eat

Consuming adequate macro- and micronutrients, staying well hydrated, and utilizing meal timing to support performance and recovery are important aspects of nutrition for dancers. However, in the hierarchy of nutrition needs, the most critical priority is adequacy (aka eating enough). Let's discuss how dancers can tell if they are eating enough (vs. too little or too much).

How Many Calories?

You may have noticed that this book does not discuss how many calories dancers need. As mentioned in the last chapter, numbers-based nutrition does not help nourish a healthy relationship with food and can be an especially problematic approach for dancers. In addition, calorie needs are highly individual and vary based on age, sex, activity level, genetics, body size, medical conditions, metabolism, and more. Without having the necessary details to tailor caloric recommendations (which would still be only an estimate), any targets provided would not be appropriate for most dancers. Assessing the benefits vs. risks of sharing calorie information can only be done in a more individual setting; therefore, I have chosen not to provide it here.

I will address some common misconceptions related to calories. The idea that we can control our body size by precisely calculating and manipulating "calories in/calories out" is an inaccurate representation of how the body works. Humans have a beautifully complex regulation system that affects how our body responds to changes in energy intake and expenditure.[49] These control mechanisms involve the brain, hormones, and metabolic shifts and are influenced by individual factors that are out of our control (i.e., our genetics).[49,50] This is why eating fewer calories doesn't always lead to weight loss and eating more calories doesn't always lead to weight gain.

It's also important to note that caloric estimates (e.g., on food labels and menus,[51,52] calculated by apps and devices,[53,54] and our own estimation of how much we eat[55–57]) are highly likely to be inaccurate. So, if the calculations that tell us how many calories we need, consume, and burn are often wrong, how beneficial is it to have this information or track it? We must also consider the mental, emotional, and quality-of-life impacts of counting and tracking calories. In addition, eating based on rules and restrictions (e.g., calorie goals) will interfere with dancers' ability to intuitively regulate their intake.[58]

Too Little/Too Much

Under-fueling is far too prevalent in dancers. The signs/symptoms of not eating enough and factors that contribute to it in dancers were covered in detail in Act I. What about overeating? Overeating is eating more than the body needs, usually resulting in uncomfortable fullness.[59] As discussed in Chapter 3, overeating is not the same as binge eating. Occasional overeating is normal and shouldn't be pathologized. However, if overeating becomes a frequent pattern, it's important to address.

First, we need to distinguish between true and perceived overeating. Do dancers (or those who train and care for them) believe they are overeating because they eat more than their peers or more than they think they "should"? Do they believe they are eating too much because their body is larger than "ideal" or because they are gaining weight? None of these factors necessarily means that a dancer is overeating. They may have greater nutrition needs than their peers, and they might need to eat more than what dance and diet culture deems appropriate. A higher weight and/or weight gain may be necessary for their body to function optimally.

The perception of overeating may come from experiencing uncomfortable fullness, which can also be a consequence of under-fueling. For example, when a dancer doesn't eat enough during the day, their very smart body that is wired for survival will typically respond with ravenous hunger that leads to eating past comfortable satiety. This is not eating more than the body needs, but rather the body making up for not having its needs met earlier. In addition, if a dancer has been routinely under-fueling, they may feel overly full with moderate portions; however, this is a sign that the dancer needs more, not less, nutrition.

In my experience, dancers are generally much more likely to undereat than to regularly consume more than their body requires. I have found that in most cases when overeating does occur, it is related to prior periods of under-fueling or some other form of restriction. There may be actual food restriction (e.g., due to dieting, disordered eating, food insecurity) or it may be more of a mental restriction. For instance, if a dancer eats a food they consider "bad" and judges themselves for it ("What's wrong with me? Why did I eat those cookies?") or sets limits on when or how much they can have in the future ("I won't eat a cookie again until next week and no more than one!"), this creates a deprivation mindset, which contributes to feeling out of control with food and overeating.

Overeating may also happen if dancers are using food as a coping mechanism, but even then, I find that there are usually restrictive behaviors or thoughts at play. We need to understand the full picture before making nutrition recommendations, and it's critical to not use a restrictive approach to try to manage overeating. The best way to prevent and address overeating is to help dancers fuel consistently and adequately and nourish a healthy and peaceful relationship with food.

The Well-Nourished Dancer

How can dancers know if they are fueling their body well without focusing on calories? The amount dancers need to eat is not static—what, when, and how much a dancer eats should shift based on their changing needs (e.g., dancers need to eat more when they are dancing more). Ideally, dancers would have access to a dietitian who can evaluate their intake, provide nutritional guidance, and help them build nourishing and adaptive eating habits.

Tuning in to hunger and fullness cues can also help dancers learn how to best nourish their body, but as mentioned in Chapter 5, most dancers benefit from using a combination of intuitive and strategic eating. Those who have been dieting or under-fueling may need to rely primarily on structured eating for some time before hunger/fullness cues become more accurate. Of note, hunger levels don't always increase in response to higher activity.[60] To prevent dancing in an energy deficit, dancers need a fueling plan that doesn't depend exclusively on hunger. (See the *Intuitive Eating* resources in the Appendix if you'd like to learn more about using the hunger/fullness scale.)

Indicators of being well nourished are often the opposite of being underfueled. Although there are medical and mental health conditions that may impact the below signs and symptoms (e.g., attention-deficit/hyperactivity disorder [ADHD], mood or digestive disorders), generally, a dancer is likely to be well fueled if:

• They have enough energy to do everything they need and want to do—dance, go to school, work, socialize, etc.

- Their body is functioning well. They have normal digestion, menstrual cycles, vital signs, and good bone health. They sleep well and have good focus and concentration. If they get sick or hurt, they recover in a reasonable amount of time.
- Their strength, stamina, and dancing improve as expected.
- Their mood is relatively stable (vs. experiencing volatility or increased anxiety, irritability, depression, etc.).
- Food thoughts take up an appropriate amount of mental space (vs. being preoccupied with food).
- Eating feels peaceful and neutral (vs. stressful and negative).

Because dancers are taught to push through discomfort and pain, they learn to ignore important signals from their body, including those that convey the need for food, hydration, and rest. At times, this is a necessary part of being a dancer. And it also creates disconnection from the body that makes it harder to recognize and respond to symptoms of under-fueling. In my work with dancers, I often find that it is only once dancers are eating better that they realize how different they feel compared to the under-fueled state to which they had become accustomed. Once they are well nourished, they are able to feel the distinction between thriving and merely surviving.

Table 6.3 Indications of Potentially Unhealthy Eating Beliefs and Behaviors

Major food group(s) and/or favorite foods are eliminated
Diet doesn't provide needed nutrients (or numerous supplements are required)
Feelings of deprivation
Required to spend more time, money, or energy on food than they have available
Following a diet because it's a current trend or influencer endorsed
Following rules that don't make sense for dancers (e.g., not eating after 7 pm, not eating any processed foods)
Requirements and/or rules are rigid and difficult to follow
Going on/off the plan (e.g., having "cheat" days)
Judging and ignoring their body's signals
Feeling anxiety, stress, and fear related to food and eating
Feeling good when they stick to the plan and feeling shame and guilt when they don't
Experiencing unpleasant physical symptoms (e.g., nausea, headache, fatigue) or feeling more depleted or down
Spending much of their time thinking about food/eating
Diet/eating habits interfere with doing things they enjoy and that are important to them

Nourishing a Healthy Relationship with Food

The influence of diet and dance culture can make it challenging for dancers to decipher between attitudes and behaviors that are beneficial and those that aren't. Table 6.3 lists some indications that a dancer's eating habits and/or relationship with food may not be healthy for them.

In contrast, what does a healthy relationship with food look like? It's eating in a way that is nourishing and enjoyable. It's eating in a way that enhances health and performance. And it's highly individual. Here are some questions for dancers to consider (ideally, the answer would be yes to all of them):

Does It Make Sense? Does the way you are eating make sense given your environment, lifestyle, resources, and preferences?

Is It Based on Good Science? Is there good evidence to support the diet's benefits for your specific needs (e.g., gluten-free diet for celiac disease)?

Is It Flexible and Sustainable? Can you imagine eating this way on holidays, vacations, and in social situations? Can you see yourself eating this way long term?

Does It Improve Body Trust? Are you able to respect and honor your body's cues?

Does It Enhance Your Health? Do you feel good physically and mentally? Does the way you are eating support a peaceful and positive relationship with food and your body?

What Dancers Find Helpful

I interviewed dancers from various genres in different stages of their careers and asked what they have found to be most helpful in terms of nutrition and fueling and what they would tell their younger selves (i.e., what they know now that they wish they knew then). Some consistent themes emerged including the importance of learning and honoring what works best for them, getting help from trusted and qualified professionals, and the need for balance. A few of the responses from these interviews are shared below. The dancers' names (anonymous, initials, or full name) and descriptions (gender, dance style, etc.) are presented according to their preferences.

> *Every body is different and one must figure out what works for theirs. ... Learning and acknowledging that there is no one-size-fits-all approach to nutrition has helped me to disregard the constant barrage of supposed advice and messaging that we are flooded with and listen to my body and my dietitian to best meet my individual needs.*
>
> *~female modern dancer*

The most impactful thing during my journey to recovery and having a healthier relationship to food and fueling myself has been to find professional help with someone I have a great connection with and trust. Working with someone who understands the demands on dancers and performance athletes physically, mentally, and emotionally while also having the proper education around nutrition is invaluable. ... I've learned that I perform my best on and off the stage when I have a meal plan in place and commit to it fully ... as I've found that sometimes I can't rely on my hunger cues to appropriately fuel for the intensity of my activity. Even during lull periods, I know it's essential to fuel myself properly so that my body can recover, I can think clearly, be present and be happier overall.

~EG, female freelance ballet dancer

Stop trying to be thinner! Eat what your body craves and don't deny yourself ... but stay ... balanced. ... Your body is yours and only yours. It will tell you what you need if you listen to it. Everyone has different needs and at different stages of their lives.

~Rosie Lani Fiedelman, female modern, jazz, and Broadway dancer

I have learnt that you require a cocktail of elements in order to best fuel yourself. Sleep alone won't fuel you, nor will one good meal. It requires you to educate yourself with what works for you, sticking to a healthier outlook, and finding solutions that fit your working day and week. ... There are multiple ways you can support your mind and body throughout the day that trained nutritionists and psychologists can help you with. Do not simply follow what dancers are showing or doing on social media!

~Steven McRae, Principal Dancer with The Royal Ballet

Main Pointes

- Optimal fueling for dancers means their diet provides necessary nutrients and supports performance and recovery; is adaptable, flexible, and enjoyable; and is free of restrictive eating practices.
- Carbohydrates are the preferred fuel for most body functions and are especially important for the brain and muscles.
- Protein is essential for muscle building and repair and is a critical nutrient for recovery from training and injury.
- Fat provides an additional source of energy and is needed to help absorb fat-soluble vitamins.
- Of the three macronutrients, dancers need more carbohydrates than protein or fat.

- Calcium, vitamin D, and iron are important micronutrients for dancers that often require extra attention to ensure needs are met.
- Key micronutrients for bone health include calcium, vitamin D, magnesium, phosphorus, potassium, vitamin C, and vitamin K.
- Dancers should use a food first approach to obtain necessary micronutrients.
- Dancers' hydration status affects energy, performance, recovery from training, and injury risk.
- What dancers eat and when they eat both impact health and performance.
- Dancers can use nutrient timing during and around dance to increase energy and focus, improve recovery, and help prevent injury.
- In the hierarchy of nutrition needs, adequacy is the top priority.
- A dancer's diet and eating habits are unhealthy if they interfere with meeting their nutritional needs, disrupt a trusting relationship with food and their body, or negatively impact their physical or mental health.

Notes

In your role/relationship with dancers, how might you encourage and support optimal fueling (keeping in mind the recommendations from Chapter 5)?

Did the Nourishing a Healthy Relationship with Food section highlight any areas in your own relationship with food that may need some healing? If so, it's never too late to find peace with food and help is available.

Endnotes

* From personal interview, 2023.

† 1300 mg/day of calcium is recommended for ages 9–18 and 1000 mg/day for ages 19–50.[61]

‡ Dancers living at latitudes >35th parallel are at higher risk for vitamin D insufficiency/deficiency.[11] In the U.S., this parallel corresponds to the southern border of Tennessee.[62]

§ Darker skin provides natural sun protection. Individuals with darker skin may need three to five times more sun exposure than those with lighter skin to make the same amount of vitamin D.[15]

** e.g., the Institute of Medicine recommends 600 IU of vitamin D per day for ages 1–70 and 800 IU/day for ages above 70.[61] For individuals "at risk" for deficiency, the Endocrine Society recommends 600–1000 IU/day for ages 1–18 and 1500–2000 IU/day for ages 19+.[15]

†† Phosphorus deficiency is rare (though it may occur in individuals with severe malnutrition who develop refeeding syndrome).[63] Excessive consumption of phosphorus (e.g., due to very high protein diets, high cola intake, or excessive consumption of foods/beverages with phosphorus-containing additives), especially in the context of low calcium intake, may have a negative impact on bone health.[23,63]

‡‡ Anemia is a condition that occurs when the body doesn't have enough healthy red blood cells.[64] Anemia can result from severely depleted iron stores (i.e., in the case of iron deficiency anemia) or other causes such as blood loss or vitamin B12 deficiency.

§§ The iron intake recommendation for (non-vegetarian) females 19–50 years of age is 18 mg/day vs. 8 mg/day for males of the same age and females age 51+.[31]

*** The cause of muscle cramps is not fully understood, though dehydration, electrolyte imbalances, fatigue, or any combination of these may be possible contributing factors.[65]

††† "Excessive" is relative. Dancers who are sensitive to caffeine may experience negative side effects with even small amounts. In addition, pediatricians advise against caffeine consumption for children and recommend that adolescents keep their intake minimal.[66]

References

1. Tribole E, Resch E. *Intuitive Eating, 4th Edition: A Revolutionary Anti-Diet Approach*. 2nd ed. St. Martin's Essentials; 2020:392.

2. Wells KR, Jeacocke NA, Appaneal R, et al. The Australian Institute of Sport (AIS) and National Eating Disorders Collaboration (NEDC) position statement on disordered eating in high performance sport. *Br J Sports Med*. 2020;54(21):1247–1258. doi:10.1136/bjsports-2019-101813

3. Cataldo CB, DeBruyne LK, Whitney EN. *Nutrition and Diet Therapy*. 6th ed. Brooks Cole; 2002:912.

4. Kerksick CM, Arent S, Schoenfeld BJ, et al. International society of sports nutrition position stand: Nutrient timing. *J Int Soc Sports Nutr*. 2017;14:33. doi:10.1186/s12970-017-0189-4

5. Beck KL, Mitchell S, Foskett A, Conlon CA, von Hurst PR. Dietary intake, anthropometric characteristics, and iron and vitamin D status of female adolescent ballet dancers living in New Zealand. *Int J Sport Nutr Exerc Metab*. 2015;25(4):335–343. doi:10.1123/ijsnem.2014-0089

6. Kalniṇa L, Selga G, Sauka M, Randoha A, Krasovska E, Lāriņš V. Comparison of body composition and energy intake of young female ballet dancers and ordinary school girls. *Proc Latv Acad Sci B Nat Exact Appl Sci*. 2017;71(6):423–427. doi:10.1515/prolas-2017-0075

7. Sousa M, Carvalho P, Moreira P, Teixeira VH. Nutrition and nutritional issues for dancers. *Med Probl Perform Art*. 2013;28(3):119–123. doi:10.21091/mppa.2013.3025

8. National Institutes of Health. Calcium fact sheet for health professionals. Accessed April 29, 2023. https://ods.od.nih.gov/factsheets/Calcium-HealthProfessional/

9. Rizzoli R. Dairy products, yogurts, and bone health. *Am J Clin Nutr*. 2014;99(5 Suppl):1256S–62S. doi:10.3945/ajcn.113.073056

10. Burckhardt P, Wynn E, Krieg M-A, Bagutti C, Faouzi M. The effects of nutrition, puberty and dancing on bone density in adolescent ballet dancers. *J Dance Med Sci*. 2011;15(2):51–60.

11. Thomas DT, Erdman KA, Burke LM. American College of Sports Medicine joint position statement. Nutrition and athletic performance. *Med Sci Sports Exerc*. 2016;48(3):543–568. doi:10.1249/MSS.0000000000000852

12. U.S. Department of Agriculture, Agricultural Research Service. FoodData Central. Accessed May 10, 2023. https://fdc.nal.usda.gov/

13. National Institutes of Health. Vitamin D fact sheet for health professionals. Accessed April 29, 2023. https://ods.od.nih.gov/factsheets/VitaminD -HealthProfessional/

14. Larson-Meyer DE, Willis KS. Vitamin D and athletes. *Curr Sports Med Rep.* 2010;9(4):220–226. doi:10.1249/JSR.0b013e3181e7dd45

15. Holick MF, Binkley NC, Bischoff-Ferrari HA, et al. Evaluation, treatment, and prevention of vitamin D deficiency: An Endocrine Society clinical practice guideline. *J Clin Endocrinol Metab.* 2011;96(7):1911–1930. doi:10.1210/jc.2011-0385

16. Wyon MA, Koutedakis Y, Wolman R, Nevill AM, Allen N. The influence of winter vitamin D supplementation on muscle function and injury occurrence in elite ballet dancers: A controlled study. *J Sci Med Sport.* 2014;17(1):8–12. doi:10.1016/j.jsams.2013.03.007

17. Giustina A, Bouillon R, Binkley N, et al. Controversies in vitamin D: A statement from the third international conference. *JBMR Plus.* 2020;4(12):e10417. doi:10.1002/jbm4.10417

18. Tardy A-L, Pouteau E, Marquez D, Yilmaz C, Scholey A. Vitamins and minerals for energy, fatigue and cognition: A narrative review of the biochemical and clinical evidence. *Nutrients.* 2020;12(1). doi:10.3390/nu12010228

19. National Institutes of Health. Magnesium fact sheet for health professionals. Accessed April 30, 2023. https://ods.od.nih.gov/factsheets/Magnesium -HealthProfessional/

20. Weaver CM, Gordon CM, Janz KF, et al. The National Osteoporosis Foundation's position statement on peak bone mass development and lifestyle factors: A systematic review and implementation recommendations. *Osteoporos Int.* 2016;27(4):1281–1386. doi:10.1007/s00198-015-3440-3

21. Benjamin RM. Bone health: Preventing osteoporosis. *Public Health Rep.* 2010;125(3):368–370. doi:10.1177/003335491012500302

22. Baxter-Jones ADG, Faulkner RA, Forwood MR, Mirwald RL, Bailey DA. Bone mineral accrual from 8 to 30 years of age: An estimation of peak bone mass. *J Bone Miner Res.* 2011;26(8):1729–1739. doi:10.1002/jbmr.412

23. Skolnik H. *The Athlete Triad Playbook.* 2020.

24. Peeling P, Blee T, Goodman C, et al. Effect of iron injections on aerobic-exercise performance of iron-depleted female athletes. *Int J Sport Nutr Exerc Metab.* 2007;17(3):221–231. doi:10.1123/ijsnem.17.3.221

25. Rosen E. Iron deficiency in athletes. August 29, 2018. Accessed May 1, 2023. https://www.gaudianiclinic.com/gaudiani-clinic-blog/2018/8/29/iron-deficiency -in-athletes

26. National Heart, Lung, and Blood Institute. Iron-deficiency anemia. March 24, 2022. Accessed May 2, 2023. https://www.nhlbi.nih.gov/health/anemia/iron -deficiency-anemia

27. Attwell C, Dugan C, McKay AKA, Nicholas J, Hopper L, Peeling P. Dietary iron and the elite dancer. *Nutrients.* 2022;14(9). doi:10.3390/nu14091936

28. Mahlamäki E, Mahlamäki S. Iron deficiency in adolescent female dancers. *Br J Sports Med.* 1988;22(2):55–56. doi:10.1136/bjsm.22.2.55

29. Sim M, Garvican-Lewis LA, Cox GR, et al. Iron considerations for the athlete: A narrative review. *Eur J Appl Physiol.* 2019;119(7):1463–1478. doi:10.1007/s00421-019-04157-y

30. Koehler K, Braun H, Achtzehn S, et al. Iron status in elite young athletes: Gender-dependent influences of diet and exercise. *Eur J Appl Physiol.* 2012;112(2):513–523. doi:10.1007/s00421-011-2002-4

31. National Institutes of Health. Iron fact sheet for health professionals. Accessed May 1, 2023. https://ods.od.nih.gov/factsheets/Iron-HealthProfessional/

32. Benardot D. Nutritional concerns for the artistic athlete. *Phys Med Rehabil Clin N Am.* 2021;32(1):51–64. doi:10.1016/j.pmr.2020.09.008
33. Ryan M. *Sports Nutrition for Endurance Athletes.* 3rd ed. VeloPress; 2012:642.
34. Li S, Fasipe B, Laher I. Potential harms of supplementation with high doses of antioxidants in athletes. *J Exerc Sci Fit.* 2022;20(4):269–275. doi:10.1016/j. jesf.2022.06.001
35. U.S. Food and Drug Administration. FDA 101: Dietary supplements. Accessed May 4, 2023. https://www.fda.gov/consumers/consumer-updates/fda-101 -dietary-supplements
36. Aschwanden C. Prohibited, unlisted, even dangerous ingredients turn up in dietary supplements. June 30, 2021. Accessed May 4, 2023. https:// www.washingtonpost.com/health/contaminated-supplements-unexpected -ingredients/2021/06/25/5d2227ec-bd62-11eb-83e3-0ca705a96ba4_story.html
37. McDermott BP, Anderson SA, Armstrong LE, et al. National athletic trainers' association position statement: Fluid replacement for the physically active. *J Athl Train.* 2017;52(9):877–895. doi:10.4085/1062-6050-52.9.02
38. American College of Sports Medicine, Sawka MN, Burke LM, et al. American College of Sports Medicine position stand. Exercise and fluid replacement. *Med Sci Sports Exerc.* 2007;39(2):377–390. doi:10.1249/mss.0b013e31802ca597
39. Armstrong LE, Ganio MS, Casa DJ, et al. Mild dehydration affects mood in healthy young women. *J Nutr.* 2012;142(2):382–388. doi:10.3945/ jn.111.142000
40. Ganio MS, Armstrong LE, Casa DJ, et al. Mild dehydration impairs cognitive performance and mood of men. *Br J Nutr.* 2011;106(10):1535–1543. doi:10.1017/S0007114511002005
41. Institute of Medicine. *Dietary Reference Intakes for Water, Potassium, Sodium, Chloride, and Sulfate.* National Academies Press; 2005. doi:10.17226/10925
42. Al-Shaar L, Vercammen K, Lu C, Richardson S, Tamez M, Mattei J. Health effects and public health concerns of energy drink consumption in the United States: A mini-review. *Front Public Health.* 2017;5:225. doi:10.3389/ fpubh.2017.00225
43. Higgins JP, Tuttle TD, Higgins CL. Energy beverages: Content and safety. *Mayo Clin Proc.* 2010;85(11):1033–1041. doi:10.4065/mcp.2010.0381
44. Committee on Nutrition and the Council on Sports Medicine and Fitness. Sports drinks and energy drinks for children and adolescents: Are they appropriate? *Pediatrics.* 2011;127(6):1182–1189. doi:10.1542/peds.2011-0965
45. Jeukendrup AE. Training the gut for athletes. *Sports Med.* 2017;47(Suppl 1):101–110. doi:10.1007/s40279-017-0690-6
46. Beelen M, Burke LM, Gibala MJ, van Loon L JC. Nutritional strategies to promote postexercise recovery. *Int J Sport Nutr Exerc Metab.* 2010;20(6):515–532. doi:10.1123/ijsnem.20.6.515
47. Burke LM, van Loon LJC, Hawley JA. Postexercise muscle glycogen resynthesis in humans. *J Appl Physiol.* 2017;122(5):1055–1067. doi:10.1152/ japplphysiol.00860.2016
48. Heaton LE, Davis JK, Rawson ES, et al. Selected in-season nutritional strategies to enhance recovery for team sport athletes: A practical overview. *Sports Med.* 2017;47(11):2201–2218. doi:10.1007/s40279-017-0759-2
49. Benton D, Young HA. Reducing calorie intake may not help you lose body weight. *Perspect Psychol Sci.* 2017;12(5):703–714. doi:10.1177/1745691617690878
50. Hall KD, Farooqi IS, Friedman JM, et al. The energy balance model of obesity: Beyond calories in, calories out. *Am J Clin Nutr.* 2022;115(5):1243–1254. doi:10.1093/ajcn/nqac031

51. Dunn R. Science reveals why calorie counts are all wrong. September 1, 2013. Accessed May 8, 2023. https://www.scientificamerican.com/article/science -reveals-why-calorie-counts-are-all-wrong/

52. Jumpertz R, Venti CA, Le DS, et al. Food label accuracy of common snack foods. *Obesity (Silver Spring)*. 2013;21(1):164–169. doi:10.1002/oby.20185

53. Banerjee P, Mendu VVR, Korrapati D, Gavaravarapu SM. Calorie counting smart phone apps: Effectiveness in nutritional awareness, lifestyle modification and weight management among young Indian adults. *Health Informatics J*. 2020;26(2):816–828. doi:10.1177/1460458219852531

54. Shcherbina A, Mattsson CM, Waggott D, et al. Accuracy in wrist-worn, sensor-based measurements of heart rate and energy expenditure in a diverse cohort. *J Pers Med*. 2017;7(2). doi:10.3390/jpm7020003

55. Carels RA, Konrad K, Harper J. Individual differences in food perceptions and calorie estimation: An examination of dieting status, weight, and gender. *Appetite*. 2007;49(2):450–458. doi:10.1016/j.appet.2007.02.009

56. Mushquash AR, Rasquinha AM, Friedman A, Ball GDC. Examining the accuracy and use of portion size estimation aids in parents of children with obesity: A randomized controlled trial. *J Nutr Educ Behav*. 2018;50(9):918–923. doi:10.1016/j.jneb.2018.06.005

57. Hernández T, Wilder L, Kuehn D, et al. Portion size estimation and expectation of accuracy. *J Food Compost Anal*. 2006;19:S14–S21. doi:10.1016/j.jfca.2006.02.010

58. Herman CP, Polivy J. The self-regulation of eating: Theoretical and practical problems. In: *Handbook of Self-Regulation: Research, Theory, and Applications*. The Guilford Press; 2004:492–508.

59. Cambridge Dictionary. Overeating. Accessed May 10, 2023. https://dictionary .cambridge.org/us/dictionary/english/overeating

60. Nattiv A, Loucks AB, Manore MM, et al. American College of Sports Medicine position stand. The female athlete triad. *Med Sci Sports Exerc*. 2007;39(10):1867–1882. doi:10.1249/mss.0b013e318149f111

61. Institute of Medicine (US) Committee to Review Dietary Reference Intakes for Vitamin D and Calcium. *Dietary Reference Intakes for Calcium and Vitamin D*. Ross AC, Taylor CL, Yaktine AL, Del Valle HB, eds. National Academies Press (US); 2011. doi:10.17226/13050

62. Wikipedia. 35th parallel north. Accessed April 29, 2023. https://en.wikipedia .org/wiki/35th_parallel_north

63. National Institutes of Health. Phosphorus fact sheet for health professionals. Accessed April 30, 2023. https://ods.od.nih.gov/factsheets/Phosphorus -HealthProfessional/

64. MedlinePlus, National Library of Medicine. Anemia. Accessed May 2, 2023. https://medlineplus.gov/ency/article/000560.htm

65. Casa DJ, DeMartini JK, Bergeron MF, et al. National athletic trainers' association position statement: Exertional heat illnesses. *J Athl Train*. 2015;50(9):986–1000. doi:10.4085/1062-6050-50.9.07

66. American Academy of Child and Adolescent Psychiatry. Caffeine and children. July 2020. Accessed May 5, 2023. https://www.aacap.org/AACAP/Families _and_Youth/Facts_for_Families/FFF-Guide/Caffeine_and_Children-131.aspx

7 Nourishing a Dancer through Injury

> *When I snapped my Achilles on the Royal Opera House Stage, I was running on empty. Not enough sleep, not enough fuel in terms of food and not mentally recharged either.*
> ~Steven McRae,* Principal Dancer with The Royal Ballet

Facing the Inevitable

Across genres, injury is a fact of life for dancers. Studies have found that in a given year (or academic year) over 80% of dancers will sustain at least one injury[1-3] and 97% experience injury at some point in their training and career.[4,5] Minor injuries may have minimal effects on a dancer's training, performance, and well-being. More severe injuries can take a heavy physical and psychological toll. Some lead to job loss or may be career-ending. Injuries that become chronic can have enduring impacts on a dancer's quality of life. Given the high rates of injury in dancers and their potentially devastating consequences, more work aimed at prevention is needed.

A necessary component of injury prevention is recognizing and working to decrease factors that contribute to their occurrence such as under-fueling, dieting, and eating disorders/disordered eating.[6] Other modifiable risk factors (within the scope of this book) include fatigue, stress, psychological distress, and poor sleep.[6-8] Several risk factors are interrelated (e.g., inadequate nutrition and fatigue, under-fueling and psychological distress) and impact both injury development and outcomes. On an individual level, identifying and addressing issues that led to a dancer's injury is critical for recovery and to prevent reoccurrence.

Preventing an injury in the first place is clearly preferable to trying to improve recovery. However, based on the above statistics, it may be overly optimistic to expect that injury is avoidable for most dancers. Therefore, dancers need to know how to best care for themselves when an injury occurs, and those who train and care for dancers need to know how to support them through what is often a difficult and scary time.

Injuries generally don't just impact an isolated body part; they affect the whole dancer. Recovery needs to focus on the whole dancer as well. To

DOI: 10.4324/9781003366171-10

support a holistic approach, this chapter includes recommendations from psychotherapists and physical therapists who specialize in working with dancers. I also interviewed dancers about their experiences with injury to learn what they found to help and hinder recovery. Quotes from these dancers[†] are interspersed throughout the chapter. Although injuries can be physically and emotionally challenging, they also present an opportunity for dancers to learn, adjust, and emerge stronger and more resilient on the other side.

Optimizing Nutrition for Healing

The most important nutrition strategy for injury prevention and recovery is ensuring that dancers are eating a balanced diet that provides enough energy (calories) and nutrients. Whether a dancer is dealing with a minor injury like a cut or bruise or a far more serious injury requiring surgery, inadequate intake of energy, carbohydrates, protein, fat, vitamins, or minerals can impair healing. Ideally, dancers have been practicing good fueling habits long before they get injured because recovery will usually be easier for a well-nourished dancer than for an under-fueled dancer.

Nutrition guidance to improve dancers' health and performance and decrease risk of injury was discussed in Chapter 6, most of which applies to injury healing as well. The next sections provide additional recommendations more specific to injury with a focus on interventions to minimize muscle loss, support tissue repair, manage inflammation, and facilitate the regain of strength and function.[9,10] The goal is to utilize nutrition to enhance recovery to help dancers heal as quickly as possible and get back to doing what they love.

Eating Enough

> *I dislocated my knee a couple years ago, and my recovery was prolonged because I didn't fuel myself correctly and I overworked my body when it wasn't ready. My injury was a result of my anorexia, and when I couldn't dance, I was terrified that I would gain weight. I barely ate and did my physical therapy exercises obsessively [which] … caused the recovery to move backwards. My recovery was supposed to take 6 weeks—it ended up being 6 months.*
>
> *~female ballet dancer*

Consuming enough energy to support injury recovery is crucial. Unfortunately, many dancers decrease their intake excessively when injured—often in an effort to prevent weight gain, though other factors also contribute to under-fueling (e.g., misconceptions about energy needs, lack of structure leading to missed meals and snacks, low appetite). Rather than helping dancers "stay in shape" to return to dance faster, negative energy balance increases muscle loss, slows down the healing process, and may prolong or prevent full recovery from the injury.[9–11] To support healing, it's preferable for dancers to err on the side of consuming a bit more than they need instead of less than they need.[9]

Activity levels typically decrease (sometimes substantially) during an injury, and dancers may mistakenly assume they don't need to eat much if they aren't dancing. Even though the energy expended in exercise might be reduced, the amount of energy the body uses at rest (i.e., basal metabolic rate) increases with injury.[10] The body requires energy to do the work of repair and healing, and the more severe the injury, the more energy that's needed for these functions.[9,11]

The amount a dancer needs to eat while injured will depend on their nutritional status prior to injury, the type and severity of injury, treatment course, and activity, among other individual factors. Depending on their circumstances, injured dancers may require less, the same amount, or more energy than they did before the injury. For example, the energy demands of recovering from major surgery and walking with crutches can be quite high.[10,11] A dancer with low energy availability prior to injury needs to eat enough to recover from the energy deficiency plus the injury. Dancers' nutrition needs will also change during the recovery process (e.g., through different phases of healing, as they advance in physical therapy). If possible, it's recommended that dancers consult with a dietitian who specializes in working with dancers to help them develop a personalized nutrition plan that will best support each stage of their recovery.

Carbohydrate Considerations

Muscle atrophy is a concern during injury, especially with immobilization and disuse.[9] Loss of muscle mass and strength will be exacerbated if muscle needs to be broken down to be used for fuel. Consuming enough carbohydrates is critical during injury so protein can be spared to do its essential jobs of repairing and rebuilding. In addition, inadequate carbohydrate intake may negatively impact bone health and healing.[12,13]

Although carbohydrate requirements *may* decrease during injury, it's generally not to the degree that dancers expect. The amount of carbohydrates that a dancer needs and how much this differs from their pre-injury intake will depend on how well fueled they were prior to injury as well as their activity level before and during injury. For dancers with significant decreases in activity, appropriate reductions in carbohydrate intake often happen naturally due to less hunger and the elimination of during-dance fueling. Drastic restriction of carbohydrates is unnecessary and will impede recovery.

When possible, it's beneficial for dancers to choose carbohydrate sources with high nutrient density such as whole grains, starchy vegetables, fruit, milk, and yogurt to enhance healing. However, dancers with low appetite and/or who are having a hard time meeting their nutrition needs should be cautious with consuming high amounts of fiber which may interfere with adequate fueling by contributing to early satiety and decreased absorption of some nutrients.

Prioritizing Protein

Getting enough high-quality protein should be a top priority for injured dancers. Three key recommendations regarding protein intake to improve recovery are:

1. **Extra**: Protein needs increase with injury, and meeting these higher requirements is crucial to help repair tissues and minimize muscle loss.[10] Most dancers will not require supplements (e.g., protein powder, protein-fortified foods) to meet protein needs during injury, but they may be helpful for dancers who find it challenging to consume enough protein.
2. **Evenly spaced**: Spacing protein consumption evenly throughout the day optimizes muscle protein synthesis (i.e., the building of new muscle tissue) and helps prevent the loss of muscle.[9]
3. **Rich in leucine**: Focusing on protein sources that are rich in the amino acid leucine may be particularly beneficial for recovery due to its role in stimulating muscle protein synthesis.[10] Good sources of leucine include meat, poultry, fish, eggs, dairy products, whey protein, tofu/soy, and beans/lentils, although plant proteins generally have less (or less absorbable) leucine than animal sources.[14,15]

Focusing on Fat (Type)

Fat provides essential components of cell membranes and energy for healing.[10] The types of fat consumed while injured deserve some attention. To support recovery, it's beneficial for dancers to select fat sources that are high in omega-3 fatty acids (found in fatty fish, ground flaxseeds, flaxseed oil, chia seeds, walnuts) and monounsaturated fatty acids (found in olive oil, canola oil, avocado, nuts/nut butter), which both have anti-inflammatory effects.[10,16] There is preliminary evidence suggesting that omega-3 fatty acids in fish oil may help reduce muscle loss during injury, but more studies are needed before routine supplementation should be recommended for dancers.[11,17]

Inflammation: It's Not All Bad

When a dancer gets injured, one of the first things that happens is their body initiates an inflammatory response.[11] Although we often think of inflammation as undesirable and something to get rid of, acute inflammation in the early stages of recovery is an essential part of the healing process.[10] Therefore, aggressive interventions to eliminate inflammation during this crucial initial phase (which can last from hours to a week depending on type and severity of injury) may be counterproductive.[11,18]

Typical dietary intake of foods with anti-inflammatory properties (e.g., fatty fish) is unlikely to be deleterious to healing.[19] However, pharmacological doses, especially in supplement form, should usually be avoided early in injury.[9] On the other hand, minimizing inflammation if it is excessive, prolonged, or chronic is important for recovery.[10] In these situations, higher intakes of anti-inflammatory compounds (e.g., fish oil, curcumin) may have a potential benefit, but more research is needed to determine their effectiveness in injured dancers and the appropriate dosage.[20,21] Given the potential for negative side effects, dancers should consult with their physician or dietitian prior to taking any supplements.

Micronutrients and More

Adequate intake of the vitamins and minerals covered in Chapter 6 is also needed to support recovery. Additional micronutrient considerations and potential nutrition interventions that may be beneficial for healing are discussed below. Although getting enough nutrients is critical, consuming excessive amounts has not been found to offer additional benefits[11,22] and may be detrimental. A food first approach to optimizing nutrition is preferable to relying on multiple supplements.

Calcium and Vitamin D

Calcium and vitamin D are critical for bone healing. Vitamin D also plays a role in regenerating muscle after injury,[23] and low vitamin D has been found to impair muscle strength recovery after knee surgery.[24] Dancers with stress fractures and other bone injuries may benefit from consuming more calcium than recommended in Chapter 6. Intakes of 1500–2000 mg/day of total calcium have been suggested,[25,26] but dancers should check with their treatment team for specific recommendations, especially prior to taking calcium supplements. Spreading calcium intake out throughout the day is a helpful strategy to maximize absorption (i.e., keep intake to no more than 500–600 mg of calcium at one time).

Vitamin D recommendations should be guided by a dancer's vitamin D status (determined with a blood test). Dancers with vitamin D insufficiency/deficiency will likely require supplementation. There remains some debate about optimal vitamin D levels for athletes.[27] As discussed in Chapter 2, the Female and Male Athlete Triad Coalition recommends a minimal level of 32 ng/mL.[28,29] If a dancer's levels are sufficient, vitamin D supplements are unnecessary.

Vitamin C and Collagen

Vitamin C has multiple functions that are vital to injury recovery including its work as an antioxidant and its essential roles in collagen synthesis and wound healing. Collagen is needed to make, maintain, and repair connective tissue such as bones, tendons, and ligaments.[30,31] You may be wondering if collagen supplements could help with injury healing, especially given their current popularity. The short answer is that there isn't enough evidence in dancers or athletes to say if collagen supplementation enhances connective tissue repair.[32] However, results from a recent review suggest that there may be a possible benefit for improving joint pain and function, particularly when used as part of a rehabilitation program, though it may take at least three months of collagen supplementation to see improvement.[30]

Because vitamin C is necessary for collagen synthesis, some collagen supplements used in research and on the market have added vitamin C. Adequate vitamin C can easily be obtained from food, and there is no evidence that increasing vitamin C consumption offers additional benefits if intake is already sufficient[22] (and, as discussed in Chapter 6, excessive vitamin C supplementation may impair performance). More research is needed to determine efficacy, optimal dosage and protocols for use, and possible contraindications of taking collagen.[33] Nonetheless, the risk of supplementing with collagen or gelatin (a form of collagen) seems relatively low.[21] It's important to note that collagen supplements and gelatin are animal-derived and therefore not vegan/vegetarian-friendly. The palatability of these products may also be a barrier to consumption. Dancers who are considering taking collagen are directed to the references cited in this section to learn more and are encouraged to discuss the pros and cons of supplementation with their treatment team.

Vitamin A, Copper, and Zinc

Other important micronutrients during injury include vitamin A, copper, and zinc, which have roles in tissue repair and wound healing and also have antioxidant functions that support recovery. Table 7.1 lists their sources.

Table 7.1 Micronutrients and Antioxidants to Support Healing

Micronutrient	Food Sources[a]
Vitamin A	Sweet potatoes, pumpkin, spinach, carrots, cantaloupe, red peppers, mango, milk (whole or fortified reduced fat/skim)
Vitamin E	Nuts, seeds, vegetable oils (e.g., sunflower, safflower), spinach, avocado
Copper	Oysters, crab, potatoes, cashews, sunflower seeds, dark chocolate, tofu, chickpeas
Zinc	Oysters, crab, shrimp, red meat, turkey, oats, fortified cereals, pumpkin seeds, lentils
Polyphenols	Tart cherries, blueberries, blackberries, raspberries, pomegranate, red grapes, apples, onions, green leafy vegetables

[a]Adapted from National Institutes of Health[34-37] and the Australian Institute of Sport.[38]

Antioxidants

The body's response to injury is a delicate balance—like so many things in life! When a dancer gets injured, inflammation and free radicals are generated and serve crucial functions in the repair process; however, if either becomes excessive, healing may be impaired.[11,39,40] Antioxidants aid recovery by protecting against damage from oxidative stress (i.e., when free radical production overwhelms the body's neutralizing capability[41]) and too much inflammation.

Polyphenols are a group of phytochemicals with antioxidant and anti-inflammatory properties that may be helpful for dancers to include in their diet to support healing.[20,42] Vitamin E is another micronutrient with antioxidant functions that is key during injury. See Table 7.1 for sources of polyphenols and vitamin E. Dancers are encouraged to consume an antioxidant-rich diet, not to take antioxidant supplements.

Timing Matters

Both *what* dancers eat and *when* they eat are important considerations during injury. Even without the structure of daily classes and rehearsals, dancers should continue to focus on nutrient timing to help improve and accelerate recovery.[10] Recommendations to support healing include:

- Eat balanced meals and snacks consistently throughout the day. Aim to have the first meal/snack within one hour of waking and then about every three to four hours.
- Include protein in every meal and snack, preferably a source high in leucine.
- Have a protein-rich snack prior to sleep.[9]
- Fuel strategically around physical therapy/rehabilitation sessions. Consuming carbohydrates and protein 15–45 minutes before therapy and additional protein within 30 minutes after therapy has been suggested as a strategy to improve outcomes.[10]

What to Avoid

Thus far we have focused on nutrients to include when dealing with an injury. There are also certain things that are beneficial to avoid. Fad diets and unnecessary food restrictions are never a good idea for dancers and can be particularly harmful during injury. Restrictive eating can lead to nutrient deficiencies, increase stress and anxiety, and harm a dancer's relationship with food and their body, all of which negatively impact recovery. Dancers should also be cautious with their use of supplements (e.g., vitamins, minerals, herbal supplements). Ensuring nutritional adequacy is critical, and for some dancers, supplements may be needed to correct deficiencies. However, taking unnecessary or excessive supplements may be detrimental for healing and/or a dancer's health.[11,21] Finally, alcohol consumption should be limited or ideally avoided during recovery because alcohol can impair muscle protein synthesis and wound healing.[17]

Caring for the Whole Dancer

As mentioned at the beginning of this chapter, injury doesn't just affect a dancer physically. Injury can be stressful and traumatic. It can bring feelings of loss, depression, anxiety, anger, fear, and shame.[43,44] Injury can threaten a dancer's livelihood and identity. And injury can exacerbate or be the catalyst for body dissatisfaction, disordered eating, or an eating disorder.[45]

Although physical and mental health are often thought of and addressed separately, the two are vitally linked (i.e., mental health directly impacts physical health and vice versa). During injury, factors such as stress and psychological distress are important to assess for and address because they not only affect dancers' health and well-being but can also influence injury outcomes.[6] According to Julie Daugherty, Company Physical Therapist for American Ballet Theatre, "The body can heal well if you give it a chance … but you have to give the body time and the proper resources—good nutrition, sleep, mental health and physical health." Figure 7.1 illustrates important aspects of injury recovery, several of which are discussed in more detail in the sections below as well as in Chapter 9.

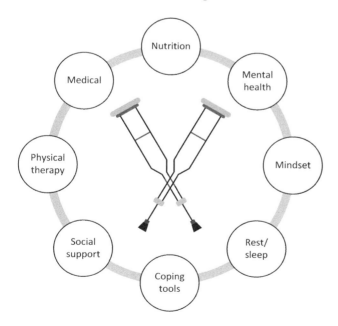

Figure 7.1 Important Aspects of Injury Recovery for Dancers.

Created by the author (image credit: Rvector/shutterstock.com).

Coping with Injury

What dancers think and how they feel about their injury and what they do in response affects their recovery. These cognitive, emotional, and behavioral aspects of how dancers react vary based on the type of injury, severity, and individual factors such as the dancer's temperament, resources, and co-occurring medical or mental health issues.[43] Approaches that can help dancers better cope with injury include acceptance of uncomfortable or painful feelings; increasing behaviors that are conducive to healing (e.g., adequate nutrition and rest, use of adaptive coping tools); and reframing negative thoughts and expectations.

Facing the Feelings

> *I've definitely been depressed when I've been injured. I think that it's healthy to process those emotions because they are real and need to be acknowledged but then they have to be released. The longer I hold on to that sadness, the harder it has been to recover emotionally. … I just try not to let the down times take over, I acknowledge them, and then I work through them.*
> ~Rosie Lani Fiedelman, female modern, jazz, and
> Broadway dancer

Mental health professionals agree with the importance of facing the difficult feelings that accompany injury. Josh Spell, licensed clinical social worker and consulting therapist for Pacific Northwest Ballet School and Company, says:

> Looking at an injury through the lens of grief has been very helpful for dancers. There are complex emotions along the way to acceptance. Anger at one's body and sadness for missing out can interrupt the path to acceptance if space has not been carved out for these emotions. Once dancers have moved towards the physical and metaphorical pain, they have a much better chance to gain true perspective and see the injury's role as a teaching moment in their career.

Self-compassion goes hand in hand with acceptance. Dancers may experience a host of negative thoughts and feelings as they deal with stresses brought on by injury (e.g., financial strain if they are unable to work and don't have paid time off, managing daily activities with limited mobility, uncertainty about their future). Rather than fighting these thoughts/feelings or judging themselves for having them, dancers can show themselves kindness and understanding, recognize that these are "normal" and expected reactions to injury, and be mindful to not become defined or consumed by negative thoughts/feelings.

Coping Tools

Effective coping strategies can help dancers deal with the stress and psychological distress of injury and improve recovery.[6,44,46] On the other hand, dancers who are not equipped with healthy coping tools may turn to maladaptive and self-harming behaviors to cope (e.g., alcohol or substance misuse, disordered eating, ignoring pain/injury) that negatively impact health, well-being, and healing.[44,46] In terms of food and eating-related coping, dancers (and those who train and care for them) need to be cautious that a desire to optimize nutrition and feel a greater sense of control over the injury doesn't lead to food rigidity, restriction, or an unhealthy relationship with food. It's also important to recognize that seeking comfort from food is normal and shouldn't be pathologized. Food is a source of pleasure and connection, which dancers may be in great need of during injury. However, there is a difference between eating emotionally with attunement, intention, and mindfulness and eating in a way that is disconnected from one's body and true physical and emotional needs.

According to Philippa Ziegenhardt, a qualified Counsellor and the former School Counsellor for The Australian Ballet School, dance is often the primary means through which dancers have four key needs met. Dance provides a physical outlet, creative outlet, sense of accomplishment, and connection. During injury, Ziegenhardt says it's important for dancers to meet these needs in alternative ways such as finding forms of movement they can still do safely and comfortably, different avenues of self-expression, other sources of achievement, and ways to stay socially connected.

There is evidence that using a combination of targeted coping tools such as relaxation techniques, imagery, and positive self-talk may shorten injury duration in dancers.[47] Other coping skills that may help dancers during recovery include mindfulness, meditation, and goal setting.[44] It's beneficial for dancers to learn and trial multiple strategies to build a "toolbox" of skills that work best for them.

Getting Support

When I was injured, I was in a very dark place, and I honestly didn't do anything right. … But knowing what I know now, I wish I had reached out to a nutritionist and a therapist to help me through that difficult time. These are valuable resources that I am lucky to have. I know that if I get injured again, my recovery process will be better with them helping me get through it.

~female ballet dancer

I use my recovery time to reconnect with people, whether it's phone calls, coffee dates, or even traveling to see family or friends. Spending time with them refuels my spirit!

~Rosie Lani Fiedelman

The quotes from these two dancers highlight the value of professional and social support. Working with a dietitian, therapist, and physical therapist (ideally who specialize in caring for dancers) helps better manage the physical and mental aspects of injury and enhances recovery. Friends, family, and dance peers and educators can be instrumental in lifting dancers' spirits and decreasing stress and feelings of isolation that accompany injury.[46] Social support can include doing fun, non-dance activities together, providing a listening ear and validation, or encouraging the dancer to get needed rest.[43] Dancers with limited mobility may need additional support with shopping, cooking, preparing meals, and transportation. Receiving support from one's "dance family" is especially important for dancers dealing with an injury while living away from home.

Rest: A Key Ingredient for Recovery

Emotionally, I find it helpful to keep working physically, having a feeling of moving forwards. ... but also realizing at times the need for rest and recovery. I pride myself on being smart with the balance between rest and pushing the body to move forwards.
                                    ~Evan Schwarz, male contemporary dancer

I believe that stress and anxiety impeded my recovery from multiple injuries. I believe that this is a multifaceted issue that stems from the deep-seated messaging that missing one class, taking any time off, and not continuing to push through pain will hinder one's improvement/ performance in dance and constitute "laziness." For me, this mentality led to a resistance to rest, which I am sure prevented tissues from healing as they could have. ... On a psychosomatic level, I think that the stress of worrying about how taking time off would affect me was probably not conducive to healing.
                                    ~female modern dancer

I find that many dancers struggle to give themselves permission to rest. They think they don't deserve it, or it's a waste of time, or that it's lazy. Dancers may see even less value in resting when they face internal and/or external pressures to return from injury. However, getting adequate rest and sleep are essential for healing. We need to help dancers find the balance between engaging in safe and supportive movement and giving their bodies sufficient time to rest so they can recover.

Caring for the Body in a Culture of Pain Tolerance

Messages about pain and rest that dancers are exposed to contribute to beliefs and behaviors that increase injury risk and impede recovery. Two recent surveys found that dancers routinely do not tell their teachers or employers when they are in pain or injured, and many delay or forgo seeking medical care.[4,48] There are numerous reasons why dancers may not reveal pain/injury and why they choose to dance through it. The dance world teaches dancers that this is expected of them. They may fear losing a role or job or feel intimidated by their teachers/choreographers/ directors.[48] They may feel pressured to perform or worry that they'll be viewed as unreliable[49] or lacking commitment.

Dancers also become accustomed to the denial of pain and discomfort. They may not be aware of or may dismiss the potentially devastating consequences of ignoring pain/injury (e.g., developing chronic pain, doing irreparable damage, shortening their career).[50] Dancers may not know how to identify pain that requires medical care and/or dance modifications.[5] Or they may be able to differentiate between different types of pain yet still choose to dance through "bad pain."[50]

Pain is a part of being a dancer, and dancers don't need to tell their teachers or employers about every ache and pain they experience or stop dancing any time they feel discomfort. Pain is also an important signal that something may be wrong, and ignoring it can cause or worsen an injury.[43] As Andrea Zujko, physical therapist and Clinic Manager at Westside Dance Physical Therapy, states, "Addressing injuries sooner rather than later will always lead to better outcomes."

Much like with eating disorders and under-fueling, a culture of acceptance is a barrier to early identification and treatment, which are critical to minimize the negative physical, psychological, and long-term impacts of injury. Dancers need to be taught how to identify pain that warrants intervention, and they need an environment that is conducive to healing. We need to create a dance culture where dancers feel safe and supported in revealing that they are in pain or injured, where they are encouraged to seek medical care, and where their health is valued and prioritized by the dancers themselves and by their dance school/company.

Learning from Injury and Emerging Stronger

I have had many injuries over the years and the most important thing that I have learned ... is that an injury is a chance to rediscover how to move. The recovery process is a way to re-teach yourself how to land or jump or whatever it is that the body parts need to do.

~Rosie Lani Fiedelman

I had to reeducate myself completely about body image, nutrition and what I believe to be a healthy body as opposed to what the traditional dance culture had told me was the "ideal" body. I also began to question the way we work as dancers and have now altered my working week to protect my body and mental health.

~Steven McRae

It can be hard for dancers to see past all the negative aspects of injury, but as the above quotes show, there are positive outcomes that can arise from injury as well. Viewing injury as a learning experience can bolster morale, reduce stress, and improve recovery.[44] Injury may reveal ways in which a dancer's mindset, beliefs, and behaviors may not be supporting their health or career longevity. Injury also offers an opportunity to explore interests and activities that a dancer's usual schedule doesn't allow time for and can help them cultivate an identity and sense of self-worth separate from dance. Sasha Gorrell, Licensed Clinical Psychologist in the University of California, San Francisco Eating Disorders Program, offers this advice for dancers:

> Read about dancers who came before you; take a course that intrigues you; start a new hobby; go to a museum (get wheelchair access if you need to). The world is wide, and the dance schedule can be narrow; try to reframe this injury hiatus as bonus time to explore all aspects of your personal identity and become a fuller, richer you. As if that isn't an important endeavor in and of itself, when you get back to dancing, the journey you had when injured will make you that much more compelling of an artist.

How You Can Help

In interviewing psychotherapists and physical therapists for this chapter, the recommendation to not rush recovery was given repeatedly. It's critical to give a dancer's body the time it needs to heal, which means not pushing dancers to return before they are ready or to do more than they have been cleared to do. Assure dancers that they won't be judged negatively for taking time off or modifying activity.[43] Spell notes, "Dancers have already put enough pressure on themselves to get back … as soon as possible. Adding more pressure only exacerbates the setback of the injury." In addition, Ziegenhardt advises that teachers/choreographers should "avoid displaying disappointment/distress/blame when you find out a dancer is injured as this can make it hard for a dancer to care for themselves."

Here are some more ways to support an injured dancer:

Check in: Ask how the dancer is feeling and coping with their injury. As Gorrell says:

> It's not unusual for depression to hit hard with injuries, particularly if they are prolonged or impactful on a career. Just as one would support anyone who was depressed, check up on them, keep them distracted and thinking as openly and positively as possible.

Communicate: According to Spell, it's important to "encourage communication and open dialogue about the injury journey." If possible, and with the dancer's consent, he suggests including dance educators and parents (when appropriate) in conversations with the dancer, doctor, and physical therapist to form a plan for recovery. Jessica Lassiter, a physical therapist in private practice, stresses the need to provide dancers with honest and supportive communication about their injury that considers their age/maturity, career stage, and individual needs.

Encourage a multidisciplinary, holistic approach: Ideally, a dancer's treatment team would include a physician, physical therapist, dietitian, and psychotherapist to ensure that the physical, nutritional, and emotional aspects of recovery are being tended to. Everyone caring for an injured dancer should be aware of their increased vulnerability to the development or exacerbation of disordered eating, body dissatisfaction, and psychological distress. Inquire about rest/sleep, eating patterns, body image, and mental health; reinforce the message that healing requires caring for the whole dancer; and make referrals to other providers so existing or emerging issues can be addressed.

Get to know the dancer: The dancer-practitioner relationship influences adherence to treatment recommendations, and dancers want to feel understood by their providers.[43] Knowing the dancer also helps you personalize the treatment approach, which can in turn contribute to better outcomes (vs. a one-size-fits-all approach).[44]

Keep dancers engaged: Spell recommends "[finding] ways to keep the dancer engaged … to reduce isolation and challenge the idea that a dancer is easily replaced." Their involvement should be based on what feels most supportive to the dancer. Some may find it helpful to watch classes and rehearsals, particularly if they are given a specific job that feels meaningful (e.g., assisting with rehearsal). For other dancers, observing from the sidelines may be detrimental. According to Ziegenhardt, "Teachers often want dancers to watch and learn but don't realize how traumatizing this can be for an injured dancer who just wants to join in and is worried about how much they are falling behind." For these dancers, keeping them connected outside of the studio (e.g., with an administrative project) may be preferable.

Manage expectations and celebrate progress: When discussing the expected recovery trajectory with dancers, don't share only the best-case scenario and be cautious with providing a specific timeline as this can cause frustration if their healing isn't going as anticipated. As physical therapist and owner of FlySpace Physical Therapy Marissa Schaeffer says, "It is simply impossible to tell a dancer exactly when they will get better because healing cannot be distilled into simple timeframes. Recovery is a complex interplay of many intrinsic and extrinsic factors that are unique to the individual." In addition, recovery isn't linear. There will likely be setbacks, but these offer valuable learning opportunities. Remind dancers not to compare their recovery to others' and that they will feel different as they return from injury. It's normal to lose strength, stamina, and technical gains, and with time and attuned work, dancers can usually get back to—and in many cases improve from—where they were before injury. During the recovery process, encourage dancers to acknowledge and celebrate their progress (e.g., increased range of motion, exercises getting easier), no matter how small it may seem.

Main Pointes

- Injuries affect the whole dancer, so recovery should focus on the whole dancer as well.
- Ensuring that dancers are eating a balanced diet that provides enough energy and nutrients is the most important nutrition strategy for injury prevention and recovery.
- Injured dancers may require less, the same amount, or more energy than they did before the injury.
- Consuming enough carbohydrates is critical during injury so protein can be spared to do its essential jobs of repairing and rebuilding.
- Getting enough high-quality protein should be a top priority for injured dancers.
- Calcium and vitamin D are critical for bone healing.
- Other important micronutrients during injury include vitamins A, C, and E; copper; and zinc.
- Dancers can utilize nutrient timing to help improve and accelerate recovery.
- Coping strategies, professional and social support, adequate rest and sleep, and viewing injury as an opportunity for learning are key during injury.
- Everyone caring for an injured dancer should be aware of their increased vulnerability to disordered eating, body dissatisfaction, and psychological distress.
- A multidisciplinary approach to treating injury helps ensure that the physical, nutritional, and emotional aspects of recovery are being addressed.

Notes

How do your own experiences with injury influence how you work with and support injured dancers?

After reading this chapter, would you change anything about how you've handled a personal injury or how you've supported an injured dancer?

Endnotes

* From personal interview, 2023.
† Dancers' names (anonymous, initials, or full name) and descriptions (gender, dance style, etc.) are presented according to their preferences.

References

1. van Winden DPAM, Van Rijn RM, Richardson A, Savelsbergh GJP, Oudejans RRD, Stubbe JH. Detailed injury epidemiology in contemporary dance: A 1-year prospective study of 134 students. *BMJ Open Sport Exerc Med.* 2019;5(1):e000453. doi:10.1136/bmjsem-2018-000453
2. Shah S, Weiss DS, Burchette RJ. Injuries in professional modern dancers: Incidence, risk factors, and management. *J Dance Med Sci.* 2012;16(1):17–25. doi:10.1177/1089313X201600103
3. Lee L, Reid D, Cadwell J, Palmer P. Injury incidence, dance exposure and the use of the movement competency screen (MCS) to identify variables associated with injury in full-time pre-professional dancers. *Int J Sports Phys Ther.* 2017;12(3):352–370.
4. Vassallo AJ, Pappas E, Stamatakis E, Hiller CE. Injury fear, stigma, and reporting in professional dancers. *Saf Health Work.* 2019;10(3):260–264. doi:10.1016/j.shaw.2019.03.001
5. Thomas H, Tarr J. Dancers' perceptions of pain and injury: Positive and negative effects. *J Dance Med Sci.* 2009;13(2):51–59.
6. Mainwaring LM, Finney C. Psychological risk factors and outcomes of dance injury: A systematic review. *J Dance Med Sci.* 2017;21(3):87–96. doi:10.12678/1089-313X.21.3.87
7. Russell JA. Preventing dance injuries: Current perspectives. *Open Access J Sports Med.* 2013;4:199–210. doi:10.2147/OAJSM.S36529
8. Ivarsson A, Johnson U, Andersen MB, Tranaeus U, Stenling A, Lindwall M. Psychosocial factors and sport injuries: Meta-analyses for prediction and prevention. *Sports Med.* 2017;47(2):353–365. doi:10.1007/s40279-016-0578-x
9. Giraldo-Vallejo JE, Cardona-Guzmán MÁ, Rodríguez-Alcivar EJ, et al. Nutritional strategies in the rehabilitation of musculoskeletal injuries in athletes: A systematic integrative review. *Nutrients.* 2023;15(4). doi:10.3390/nu15040819
10. Smith-Ryan AE, Hirsch KR, Saylor HE, Gould LM, Blue MNM. Nutritional considerations and strategies to facilitate injury recovery and rehabilitation. *J Athl Train.* 2020;55(9):918–930. doi:10.4085/1062-6050-550-19
11. Tipton KD. Nutritional support for exercise-induced injuries. *Sports Med.* 2015;45 Suppl 1:S93–104. doi:10.1007/s40279-015-0398-4
12. Kuikman MA, Mountjoy M, Stellingwerff T, Burr JF. A review of nonpharmacological strategies in the treatment of relative energy deficiency in sport. *Int J Sport Nutr Exerc Metab.* 2021;31(3):268–275. doi:10.1123/ijsnem.2020-0211
13. Upadhyay J, Farr OM, Mantzoros CS. The role of leptin in regulating bone metabolism. *Metab Clin Exp.* 2015;64(1):105–113. doi:10.1016/j.metabol.2014.10.021
14. Karpinski C, Rosenbloom CA. *Sports Nutrition: A Handbook for Professionals.* 6th ed. Academy of Nutrition and Dietetics; 2017:277.
15. Berrazaga I, Micard V, Gueugneau M, Walrand S. The role of the anabolic properties of plant- versus animal-based protein sources in supporting muscle mass maintenance: A critical review. *Nutrients.* 2019;11(8). doi:10.3390/nu11081825
16. Clark N. *Nancy Clark's Sports Nutrition Guidebook.* 6th ed. Human Kinetics Publishers; 2020:800.
17. Turnagöl HH, Koşar ŞN, Güzel Y, Aktitiz S, Atakan MM. Nutritional considerations for injury prevention and recovery in combat sports. *Nutrients.* 2021;14(1). doi:10.3390/nu14010053

18. Maruyama M, Rhee C, Utsunomiya T, et al. Modulation of the inflammatory response and bone healing. *Front Endocrinol (Lausanne)*. 2020;11:386. doi:10.3389/fendo.2020.00386
19. Fritsche KL. The science of fatty acids and inflammation. *Adv Nutr*. 2015;6(3):293S–301S. doi:10.3945/an.114.006940
20. Papadopoulou SK, Mantzorou M, Kondyli-Sarika F, et al. The key role of nutritional elements on sport rehabilitation and the effects of nutrients intake. *Sports (Basel)*. 2022;10(6). doi:10.3390/sports10060084
21. Maughan RJ, Burke LM, Dvorak J, et al. IOC consensus statement: Dietary supplements and the high-performance athlete. *Br J Sports Med*. 2018;52(7):439–455. doi:10.1136/bjsports-2018-099027
22. Close GL, Sale C, Baar K, Bermon S. Nutrition for the prevention and treatment of injuries in track and field athletes. *Int J Sport Nutr Exerc Metab*. 2019;29(2):189–197. doi:10.1123/ijsnem.2018-0290
23. Latham CM, Brightwell CR, Keeble AR, et al. Vitamin D promotes skeletal muscle regeneration and mitochondrial health. *Front Physiol*. 2021;12:660498. doi:10.3389/fphys.2021.660498
24. Barker T, Martins TB, Hill HR, et al. Low vitamin D impairs strength recovery after anterior cruciate ligament surgery. *J Evid Based Complementary Altern Med*. 2011;16(3):201–209. doi:10.1177/2156587211413768
25. United States Olympic & Paralympic Committee Sport Nutrition Team. Nutrients for bone/joint injury recovery. 2020.
26. Moreira CA, Bilezikian JP. Stress fractures: Concepts and therapeutics. *J Clin Endocrinol Metab*. 2017;102(2):525–534. doi:10.1210/jc.2016-2720
27. Knechtle B, Jastrzębski Z, Hill L, Nikolaidis PT. Vitamin D and stress fractures in sport: Preventive and therapeutic measures-a narrative review. *Medicina (Kaunas)*. 2021;57(3). doi:10.3390/medicina57030223
28. De Souza MJ, Nattiv A, Joy E, et al. 2014 Female Athlete Triad Coalition Consensus Statement on treatment and return to play of the female athlete triad. 1st International Conference held in San Francisco, California, May 2012 and 2nd International Conference held in Indianapolis, Indiana, May 2013. *Br J Sports Med*. 2014;48(4):289. doi:10.1136/bjsports-2013-093218
29. Fredericson M, Kussman A, Misra M, et al. The male athlete triad-A consensus statement from the Female and Male Athlete Triad Coalition Part II: Diagnosis, treatment, and return-to-play. *Clin J Sport Med*. 2021;31(4):349–366. doi:10.1097/JSM.0000000000000948
30. Khatri M, Naughton RJ, Clifford T, Harper LD, Corr L. The effects of collagen peptide supplementation on body composition, collagen synthesis, and recovery from joint injury and exercise: A systematic review. *Amino Acids*. 2021;53(10):1493–1506. doi:10.1007/s00726-021-03072-x
31. Ryan M. *Sports Nutrition for Endurance Athletes*. 3rd ed. VeloPress; 2012:642.
32. Holwerda AM, van Loon LJC. The impact of collagen protein ingestion on musculoskeletal connective tissue remodeling: A narrative review. *Nutr Rev*. 2022;80(6):1497–1514. doi:10.1093/nutrit/nuab083
33. Australian Institute of Sport. AIS sports supplement framework: Collagen. March 2021.
34. National Institutes of Health. Vitamin A and carotenoids fact sheet for health professionals. Accessed June 22, 2023. https://ods.od.nih.gov/factsheets/VitaminA-HealthProfessional/
35. National Institutes of Health. Vitamin E fact sheet for health professionals. Accessed June 23, 2023. https://ods.od.nih.gov/factsheets/VitaminE-HealthProfessional/

36. National Institutes of Health. Copper fact sheet for health professionals. Accessed June 23, 2023. https://ods.od.nih.gov/factsheets/Copper-HealthProfessional/
37. National Institutes of Health. Zinc fact sheet for health professionals. Accessed June 23, 2023. https://ods.od.nih.gov/factsheets/Zinc-HealthProfessional/
38. Australian Institute of Sport. AIS sports supplement framework: Fruit-derived polyphenols. March 2021.
39. Kozakowska M, Pietraszek-Gremplewicz K, Jozkowicz A, Dulak J. The role of oxidative stress in skeletal muscle injury and regeneration: Focus on antioxidant enzymes. *J Muscle Res Cell Motil.* 2015;36(6):377–393. doi:10.1007/s10974-015-9438-9
40. Quintero KJ, Resende A de S, Leite GSF, Lancha Junior AH. An overview of nutritional strategies for recovery process in sports-related muscle injuries. *Nutrire.* 2018;43(1):27. doi:10.1186/s41110-018-0084-z
41. Cataldo CB, DeBruyne LK, Whitney EN. *Nutrition and Diet Therapy.* 6th ed. Brooks Cole; 2002:912.
42. Sousa M, Teixeira VH, Soares J. Dietary strategies to recover from exercise-induced muscle damage. *Int J Food Sci Nutr.* 2014;65(2):151–163. doi:10.310 9/09637486.2013.849662
43. Mainwaring LM, Krasnow D, Kerr G. And the dance goes on: Psychological impact of injury. *J Dance Med Sci.* 2001;5(4):105–115. doi:10.1177/1089313X0100500402
44. Pollitt EE, Hutt K. Viewing injury in dancers from a psychological perspective – A literature review. *J Dance Med Sci.* 2021;25(2):75–79. doi:10.12678/1089-313X.061521a
45. Bratland-Sanda S, Sundgot-Borgen J. Eating disorders in athletes: Overview of prevalence, risk factors and recommendations for prevention and treatment. *Eur J Sport Sci.* 2013;13(5):499–508. doi:10.1080/17461391.2012.740504
46. Pentith R, Moss SL, Lamb K, Edwards C. Perfectionism among young female competitive Irish dancers – Prevalence and relationship with injury responses. *J Dance Med Sci.* 2021;25(2):152–158. doi:10.12678/1089-313X.061521k
47. Noh Y-E, Morris T, Andersen MB. Psychological intervention programs for reduction of injury in ballet dancers. *Res Sports Med.* 2007;15(1):13–32. doi:10.1080/15438620600987064
48. Veirs KP, Baldwin JD, Fagg A, et al. Survey of ballet dance instructors and female dancers concerning perception of dance-related pain and injury. *Orthop Pract.* 2021;33(4):226–233.
49. Jacobs CL, Cassidy JD, Côté P, et al. Musculoskeletal injury in professional dancers: Prevalence and associated factors: An international cross-sectional study. *Clin J Sport Med.* 2017;27(2):153–160. doi:10.1097/JSM.0000000000000314
50. Harrison C, Ruddock-Hudson M. Perceptions of pain, injury, and transition-retirement: The experiences of professional dancers. *J Dance Med Sci.* 2017;21(2):43–52. doi:10.12678/1089-313X.21.2.43

8 Nourishing Balanced and Resilient Body Image in Dancers

A dancer's personal vision of [their] body is an important part of [their]
psychological health and well-being, and it can help or hinder [their] dance
performance in the studio.
~Sally A. Radell and IADMS Dance Educators' Committee[1]

What Is Body Image?

Body image is your relationship with your body[2] and it encompasses several interrelated components including[3]:

- **Perceptions of your body**: how you visualize your body, how you imagine others see your body.
- **Attitudes toward your body**: your thoughts, feelings, beliefs, and evaluations of your body and what you do as a result.
- **Experience in your body**: how you inhabit your body, what it feels like to go through the world living in your body.[4]

Body image is shaped and expressed through these various aspects and can be improved through them as well. We are not born disliking our bodies. Think about a child's wonder as they discover their hands, their feet, their nose, and their joy as they learn to do new things with their body. Eventually they begin to make comparisons (e.g., your hand is bigger than my hand), but different is just different until they learn that some physical attributes are valued more than others. Sadly, the body appreciation we are born with doesn't last long. Body dissatisfaction is seen in children as young as five.[3,5]

The dance world can have a profound impact on dancers' body image, but it doesn't affect dancers in a vacuum. The way dancers see themselves, what they think and how they feel about their body, how connected they are to their body, and how they behave toward it are also influenced by internal and external factors including individual physical and psychological characteristics, age, gender, sexuality, race/ethnicity, culture, lived experiences, family, peers, media, socioeconomic status, and more.[3,6] In other words, body image is complex!

DOI: 10.4324/9781003366171-11

It's beyond the scope of this book to explore how each of the above factors and their intersections may affect a dancer's relationship with their body. However, it's essential to consider all the layers of body image and ensure we are not neglecting the experiences of dancers from more marginalized groups (e.g., non-White, non-cisgender, in a larger body, etc.). Not every dancer has a poor relationship with their body, but for those who do, there isn't a one-size-fits-all approach to improving body image. Rather, each dancer's unique circumstances and lived experience need to guide the path to healing.

Body Image Distortions

How accurately you perceive your body is one aspect of body image. It's common, and not necessarily problematic, to sense your body differently from the inside than it appears on the outside. However, for some individuals, having a distorted view of their body or appearance (e.g., misestimating body size or muscularity) can cause significant distress. Body image distortion is a feature of eating disorders.[6] When body image issues are present, it's critical to assess for eating disorders because these complex conditions, which are prevalent in dancers,[7] require specialized treatment from qualified professionals. Aside from this brief mention, this chapter will not cover body image distortions (see Chapter 3 for more information on eating disorders).

Body Image Matters

Why should dancers and the people who train and care for them be concerned with body image? Body image impacts dancers' physical and mental health, well-being, and performance. As discussed in previous chapters, body dissatisfaction is common in dancers across different genres and is a strong predictor of developing an eating disorder. Body dissatisfaction is also associated with harmful weight control behaviors, anxiety, depression, and increased inflammation. How a dancer feels about their body affects how they nourish and care for themselves. By improving how they nourish and care for themselves, dancers can also nurture better body image.

Body Image Goals

Body image is often thought of as either positive or negative, good or bad. If you aren't happy with your body, you're expected to go from disliking or even hating your body to loving every inch of it all the time. This way of thinking can be a barrier to improving body image, especially in the context of perfectionism. Not only are body ideals in diet and dance culture unrealistic and unattainable, but so are body image goals. The other problem with this framing of body image is that it makes it seem like positive body image is simply the opposite or absence of negative body image, which is inaccurate and doesn't capture the complexity of positive body image.[8] Positive body image is not defined or achieved merely by liking how you look, but rather is multi-faceted and includes active practices (e.g., body appreciation, challenging body ideals). In addition, the idea of positive body image may not resonate for some dancers—instead, body neutrality* may feel like a more attainable or worthwhile goal.

Whether aiming for more positive or neutral body image, both involve greater connection with and care for the body (vs. disconnection and neglect), as shown in Figure 8.1. For example, imagine how you would care for a young child or a toddler version of yourself. When the child cries, do you ignore them or try to figure out what need they are expressing? When the child is hungry, do you withhold food if you don't like how they look? When it's time for their nap, do you make them run around outside instead? Improving body image involves working toward a more attuned and caring relationship with your body—one where you can treat your body in a loving and respectful way, even when you feel displeased, disappointed, or let down by it. And like any other relationship, your relationship with your body requires ongoing work.

Redefining what we are striving for in terms of body image helps move us away from the notion that changing our body is the best way to feel better about our body.[†] Despite an abundance of diet culture messaging to the contrary, weight loss doesn't guarantee improved body image.[9] In the short term, body changes that bring a dancer closer to diet or dance culture's "ideal" may increase aspects of body satisfaction, especially when these body changes are met with praise or other forms of positive reinforcement. However, this also strengthens beliefs that certain bodies have more value than others and that a dancer's body determines their worth, which are counter to truly positive (or neutral) body image. And what happens when a dancer's new body can't be sustained or can only be maintained through harmful or disordered behaviors?

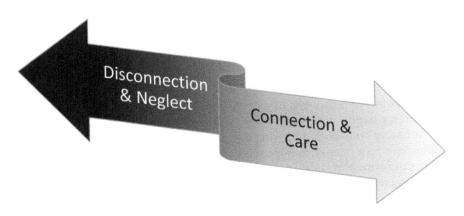

Figure 8.1 Body Image Goals: Moving Toward Greater Connection and Care.

Body size and shape play a role in body image, but having a body that meets or is close to meeting the "ideal" does not make a dancer immune to negative body image. In addition, body image is not static—it may fluctuate from day to day, moment to moment, and differ based on environment, which illustrates that body image is about so much more than the body. In most cases, the key to improving body image is changing your mindset, not your body.

The goal of helping dancers build more balanced and resilient body image recognizes that dancers are aesthetic athletes, and, therefore, expecting them not to place any importance on how their body looks is likely not realistic. At the same time, appearance should not have an outsized influence (or ideally, even a significant influence) on dancers' relationship with their body. Additionally, most dancers (along with the rest of us) will have uncomfortable or negative body moments. Dancers may not be able to fully control all the factors that affect their body image (e.g., body comments, reinforcement of the thin ideal in dance), but they can learn ways to lessen the negative impact of these forces.

Additional Considerations

A comprehensive discussion of body image would require an entire book. In fact, there are several books written on the subject (some of which I've cited). This chapter provides an introduction to several research-based concepts and practices that I and colleagues find helpful when supporting dancers in nurturing more harmony with their body image. This guidance is not intended to be used as a body image treatment manual. The way you use the information will depend on your qualifications and your role and relationship with dancers. Adequate training and experience are necessary before engaging in body image "work" with dancers.

Although this chapter will not specifically address trauma, it's critical to acknowledge the significant impact trauma can have on body image, and to commit to ensuring that body image discussions and interventions are trauma-informed. A sense of safety is paramount to body image healing. For dancers who have had experiences that contribute to a fraught relationship with their body, it may be best to get professional help to support them in addressing body image concerns.

Like in Chapter 7, I have included recommendations from dance psychotherapists and insights from dancers' lived experiences. The "Body Image in Action" prompts are offered to illustrate what covered concepts may look like in practice. I hope you will come away from this chapter seeing that negative body image is not inevitable for dancers and when it exists, it doesn't have to be permanent. It is possible to improve how dancers think and feel about, care for, and experience their bodies, and to help them begin to heal from body image injuries. And as has been a theme throughout this book, meaningful change will take contributions from all of us.

Expecting dancers to have positive (or neutral) body image while living and dancing in environments that bombard them with messages that they aren't good enough (e.g., they have the wrong body, skin color, gender) is like asking them to hike up a mountain while carrying boulders on their backs. This chapter focuses on ways to help dancers on an individual level, yet we must not lose sight of how vital it is to also foster broader change—in the dance world and beyond. Parents, peers, and dance educators have a powerful influence on dancers' body image.[10] If every person in a dancer's life adopted the practices highlighted in this chapter, it could have a huge positive ripple effect![11]

Taking Stock

Because body image has multiple elements and negative body image can manifest in different ways, it's helpful for dancers to consider their personal relationship with their body. How would they describe their body image? How does it affect them? Table 8.1 lists additional questions to promote body image self-awareness. It may be most appropriate to explore these questions with a qualified professional (e.g., therapist and/or dietitian with body image training/experience).

Dancers will likely notice that different aspects of their body image (i.e., perceptions, attitudes, and experiences) occur on a spectrum. They may sometimes feel consumed by negative body thoughts, and at other times, their thoughts may be more neutral or positive. Negative feelings about their body may sometimes lead to disordered eating or other compensatory behaviors, while other times, they may be able to tolerate the uncomfortable emotions until they pass or use healthy coping tools.

Table 8.1 Building Body Image Self-Awareness

How have your life experiences influenced your body image?
How much time/energy do you spend judging or criticizing your body, trying to change it, or worrying about what others think of your body?
How often do you think about things you like or appreciate about your body?
How often do you compare your body to others?
Does your body image get in the way of enjoying life? If yes, how so (e.g., do you avoid activities because of how you feel in your body)?
Does your body image affect your eating or exercise habits? If yes, how so?
What do you do when/if you feel bad in/about your body?
What thoughts, feelings, and/or sensations accompany uncomfortable body days? What about during times you feel more comfortable in your body?

Adapted from Cash[2] and Wood-Barcalow, Tylka, and Judge.[11]

It's valuable to identify circumstances that contribute to body image shifts. How does the way a dancer thinks, feels, and acts toward their body change in different settings (e.g., dance, school, home) or with different people? What happens when other body issues or sensations are present (e.g., digestive discomfort, premenstrual syndrome [PMS], injury)? How does their emotional state impact their body image (e.g., what happens when they are tired, anxious, or sad)?

For qualified professionals working with dancers on body image concerns, and for dancers themselves, it's important to know what dancers would like to change about their relationship with their body. What do they wish was different? Maybe they would like to spend far less time and energy criticizing themselves. Perhaps they would like to be less preoccupied with negative body thoughts so they can be more present in their relationships. Maybe they recognize how much body comparison affects them and want to decrease that behavior. Perhaps they wish they would allow themselves to eat their favorite foods on "bad" body image days. When dancers are working toward change that is meaningful to them, it provides motivation to keep going, especially as they face challenges. As dancers embark on their journey to more balanced and resilient body image, they are encouraged to bring along their trusted companion: self-compassion.

Externalizing the Problem

I would tell a younger me that the messaging of the ballet world is toxic and wrong. During my college years, I found myself brainwashed by a subset of professors who had me convinced that any part of my body that wasn't straight or flat was a problem that would interfere with my career. This damage has taken years to undo, and now I would want my younger self to have had the knowledge and self-worth to reject this dangerous notion of an "ideal dancer's body."

~female modern dancer

A dancer's body is not the problem. The problem is the system(s) that makes them believe that it is. We need to help dancers see their body image through a much wider lens—one that shows how they view, evaluate, think, and feel about their body in the context of what they've been taught and had repeatedly reinforced by diet and dance culture. As Josh Spell, licensed clinical social worker and consulting therapist for Pacific Northwest Ballet School and Company, says:

It is difficult to talk about body image without acknowledging the system that has normalized body image dissatisfaction. Reminding dancers that body image struggles are a structural problem that contribute to individual distress can help take some of the self-blame off a dancer.

Philippa Ziegenhardt, qualified Counsellor and the former School Counsellor for The Australian Ballet School, shared related sentiments. To help dancers build more positive and resilient body image, she says we have to "[educate] them about the myths and foolishness so often involved in [dancer] body biases so they have their eyes open to it and don't get as easily sucked in."

Dancers' negative views and beliefs about bodies don't start out as their own. Dancers (and the rest of us) have been exposed to messages about which bodies are deemed "good bodies" for so long that these designations become accepted as fact and what they believe as true. But constructs about what makes a body better or worse are societal inventions.[12]

Dancers did not choose or consent to the mindset that makes them feel bad about their bodies. An essential step in body image healing is for dancers to evaluate and question why they believe what they do. Who benefits from them continuing to subscribe to these beliefs? It's valuable for dancers to learn about the racist, sexist, and classist roots of diet culture and the ways in which the dance world may amplify diet culture's messages and values (see Chapter 1). Then dancers can begin to sort what beliefs are truly theirs and worth keeping and which are harmful ideas that belong to diet and dance culture and need to be let go.

Tuning In

Values

Your core values are an integral part of who you are. They are your internal compass guiding you toward a more fulfilling life. Core values include compassion, justice, creativity, making a difference, and many others. Finding ways to connect to and stay true to your values can help you through difficult times and inspire you to move toward needed change.[11] For example, if one of your core values is kindness, treating yourself cruelly by withholding food or engaging in punishing exercise when you're having an uncomfortable body day is misaligned with that value. In contrast, you can make space for your discomfort and respond with an act of kindness (e.g., feeding yourself a delicious, nourishing meal) which corresponds with your values.

Making these types of values-driven choices can help dancers improve their body image (see discussion of body image flexibility in Chapter 5). When dancers increase their connection to their values it builds a sense of self-worth separate from appearance. Aligning with their core values can help dancers reject unrealistic and harmful body standards and can help them honor their needs and their body amidst the harsh pressures and expectations of the dance world. Sasha Gorrell, Licensed Clinical Psychologist in the University of California, San Francisco Eating Disorders Program, offers this advice:

> I like to invite dancers to live in line with their values and recognize that when they see people who are very thin being favored in a way

that feels unfair, this doesn't mean they need to compromise their own health to fall in line.

Body Image in Action: What are your core values? Consider some of the values mentioned above or do an online search and you will find many different values listed. As you read through them, choose values that resonate with you and then narrow them down to your top five. Make sure they really feel like your true values and don't belong to diet or dance culture. Does the way you treat your body correspond with your values?[11] If not, what actions could you take to bring you closer to your values?

Interoception and Attunement

Think about what it feels like when you have a full bladder, or your heart is beating fast. Can you sense when your stomach is empty? What does sadness feel like in your body? Interoceptive awareness is the ability to perceive physical sensations that come from inside the body.[13] These internal signals provide essential information about your body's physical and emotional state that help get needs met[13] (e.g., when your bladder feels full, you use the bathroom).

How accurately we perceive our internal signals is important to consider as both heightened and diminished sensitivity can interfere with self-care. For example, hyposensitivity to hunger and/or hypersensitivity to fullness may contribute to under-fueling or disordered eating.[14] Research suggests that impaired interoceptive awareness and/or accuracy may predispose individuals to body image dissatisfaction and eating disorders.[15,16] Life experiences (e.g., trauma, dieting) as well as medical, mental health, and developmental conditions can affect how dancers experience and interpret their body sensations, how much they trust and value them, and how they respond (i.e., honoring their needs vs. judging/ignoring them).

Attunement—the ability to perceive, understand, and respond to your needs—is an essential component of health and well-being. Every time you honor your body's needs you build body trust. But you can't give your body what it needs if you don't know what that is. External influences and pressures can also contribute to misattunement,[17] as may be the case for many dancers. According to Ziegenhardt, "Dancers often put others' needs before their own, which makes it hard to recognize when they are having a need." She helps dancers learn how to identify when they have an unmet need and reinforces that "they are allowed to ask for their needs to be met." Spell notes, "Dancers often only check in with their bodies when they want to change something about it." He "encourage[s] dancers to check in with their bodies through regular practices to identify a variety of sensations which can be positive, challenging or neutral." In addition, he says "Describing emotions, feelings and sensations in the body through colors, imagery or temperature can also increase [dancers'] understanding of their needs."

Body Image in Action: Building self-awareness of body sensations and the needs they communicate—as well as not judging such signals/needs—facilitates attunement. Mindfulness, or "paying attention, on purpose, in the present moment, non-judgmentally,"[18] can help in both areas. Consider incorporating or increasing mindfulness practices such as breathing exercises, meditation, yoga, and body scans.[19]

Your Body, Your Home

Positive Embodiment

Catherine Cook-Cottone's description of embodiment ties together the three areas just discussed in the Tuning In section: "Embodiment reflects a developing, evolving experience of self that unfolds within the context of attunement with internal needs, a personal sense of purpose and meaning, and the external experience of self in the world."[20] A simpler way to define embodiment is "how we experience and engage our bodies in the world."[11]

Niva Piran identified five dimensions of embodiment[4] that can provide a framework to support the development of more balanced body image and promote body image healing. These five related components of embodiment occur on a continuum from positive embodiment to negative or disrupted embodiment as outlined below[4,11]:

Body Connection and Comfort

- Positive embodiment: You feel "at one" with or "at home" in your body. Your body is a comfortable vessel from which you engage with the world.
- Negative/Disrupted embodiment: You feel disconnected or separate from your body. You feel ashamed or fearful of your body or angry at it. It feels like something you need to control or fix.

Agency and Functionality

- Positive embodiment: You feel empowered to use your voice and express your opinions. You lead others. You engage in joyful movement and value what your body can do.
- Negative/Disrupted embodiment: You have a hard time voicing your opinions or feel they don't matter. You tend to follow others. You don't feel you can stand up for yourself. You engage in punishing/unenjoyable exercise for the purpose of "fixing" your body.

Experience and Expression of Desire

- Positive embodiment: You are in touch with your bodily desires (i.e., appetite, sexual desire), feel positive about the experience of having them, and respond to your desires in self-caring ways.

- Negative/Disrupted embodiment: You are disconnected from your desires or ignore or judge them.

Attuned Self-care

- Positive embodiment: You are tuned in to your body's signals and respond to them in nurturing ways to meet your physical, emotional, and relational needs.
- Negative/Disrupted embodiment: You are disconnected from your body's cues and/or neglect your needs.

Inhabiting the Body as a Subjective Site

- Positive embodiment: You inhabit your body from the inside out rather than the outside in (i.e., you resist objectification). You are critical of the preoccupation with appearance and pressures to conform to body "ideals."
- Negative/Disrupted embodiment: You experience your body as a critical observer of it. You focus more on how your body looks than how it feels. You spend a lot of time/energy trying to "fix" your body/appearance to meet "ideals."

As you read through the above aspects of embodiment, you may have thought of several ways in which the dance world can disrupt positive embodiment and may even foster negative embodiment. Embodiment is inextricably linked to social location, lived experiences, and safety.[4] I recently attended a session given by Piran at a conference and found this statement of hers especially powerful: "There is no safety within the context of inequity."[21] A dancer can't feel at peace or comfortable in a body that is under threat. We need to consider how racism, discrimination, sexual harassment, trauma, and other factors that impact dancers' sense of safety disrupt their ability to experience positive embodiment. Health challenges, chronic illness, disability, and gender dysphoria can also affect embodiment.[4]

Body Image in Action: Check in with your body in this moment. Is there anything that might make you more comfortable (e.g., a change of clothes, temperature, or position)? Is your body sending you any messages about something it needs (e.g., food, water, rest, connection, soothing)? What can you do to meet this need? These are examples of ways to increase Body Connection and Comfort and Attuned Self-care. Behaviors that can improve the other dimensions of positive embodiment include advocating for your needs and boundaries (Agency and Functionality), giving yourself permission to eat your favorite food(s) without judgment (Experience and Expression of Desire), and reducing body-checking behaviors like weighing yourself (Inhabiting the Body as a Subjective Site).

Practices to Nourish More Balanced Body Image

You need to nourish the seeds of positive (or neutral) body image if you want them to flourish. On the other hand, if you put most of your attention and energy on thoughts and behaviors that increase negative body image, that will be what grows. Self-compassion can support the development of more balanced body image and protect against negative body image.[22]

The next sections contain additional guidance to help dancers nurture a better relationship with their body. You will notice that these areas are inter-related with each other and overlap with what has been discussed in the past sections. As mentioned previously, body image "work" needs to be guided by each dancer's unique needs and circumstances. Some of the concepts listed below may not resonate with some dancers and that's okay. They don't have to adopt every suggestion—perhaps they can find one or two that feel mean-ingful and safe to try.

Body Acceptance

> *I spent much of my early years as a professional so self-conscious about my body and all of the "faults" that I had been made aware of by some coaches or teachers. I wish I was able to tell my younger self to stop wasting energy on what I think is wrong with my body. My body is mine and that's what I have to work with. It's great in its own way!*
>
> ~Steven McRae, Principal Dancer with The Royal Ballet

> *I have learned that much of my body is just genetics as I have a smaller frame and always desired to have bulkier muscles. But [now] I take pride in my strong and lengthy muscles.*
>
> ~Evan Schwarz, male contemporary dancer

> *I wish I knew that being bogged down worrying about the shape of my body was counterproductive. I wish I knew that what counted wasn't the shape of my body, but my strength, my articulation, my artistic choices, my musical-ity, my joy.*
>
> ~female modern dancer

These are three dancers' responses to my questions, "What would you tell the younger you about body image? What do you know now that you wish you knew then?" Their answers share the powerful message of the value of body acceptance. What if we could spare dancers the time and heartache of being at war with their body? They only get one body, and every dancer's body has unique qualities worth embracing.

Body acceptance may feel impossible for some dancers—"I will never love my body. I don't want to accept this body." Dancers' concept of what body acceptance means can be a barrier to embracing the practice. It would be lovely if they accepted and felt positively toward their body most of the time, but this may be too far of a leap from where they are now. Depending on the identities they hold and their lived experience, it may feel unattainable. Perhaps aiming for body neutrality or even just tolerating their body would feel more realistic, and these can be valuable steps toward greater acceptance (though ideally dancers won't settle for merely tolerating their body).

It may also be helpful to shift the idea of what body acceptance means. Body acceptance does not have to mean that you like your body or are satisfied with it. Instead, body acceptance can be thought of as:

- Accepting the influence of genetics on body size/shape (even if you wish your body were different).
- Accepting that attempts to change your body size/shape into something it isn't genetically meant to be can harm your physical and/or mental health.
- Accepting that this is the body you have today; it is the body that allows you to think, breathe, dance (and so much more!), and it is deserving of kindness, care, and respect even if you're not 100% happy with how it looks or functions.[8]
- Accepting that there is no such thing as a perfect body and you can choose to focus on your assets rather than your perceived flaws.[8]

Body Image in Action: Write down some of your body's unique characteristics that you feel positive or neutral about. Do any of your physical attributes remind you of those of your family members or ancestors?[11] If so, how does it feel to have this body connection to your heritage?[8]

Body Appreciation

> *I would tell my younger self that you only get one body, and it's a privilege that we have such a vessel to go through life with. I wish I was able to see that I am a beautiful human being no matter what that vessel looks like. I also wish I knew how lucky I am to witness my body change as I get older. As we age, our body goes through phases, and it's a luxury to get to witness that.*
>
> *~female ballet dancer*

How often do you feel thankful for what your body does for you? How often do you notice the good in your body?[11] By contrast, how many messages do you hear from society, the dance world, and yourself that make you think about all that's "wrong" with your body? By regularly and purposefully bringing attention to and acknowledging what you appreciate about your body, you can shift this balance and cultivate more positive thoughts and feelings about your body.

Focusing on gratitude for what the body is capable of doing (i.e., functionality appreciation)[11] may be an especially useful entry point to improving body image in dancers as there is so much to appreciate about what their bodies enable them to do. As Gorrell says,

> The human body is incredible and building appreciation for its capabilities (rather than what it looks like) can be a way to create a more positive and resilient body image. I like to nail home the idea that dancers are first and foremost athletes—before they are artists. ... [This] places emphasis on the activity itself, which can then inspire dancers to take care of their bodies to optimize performance (rather than aesthetics). Secondly, focusing on functional aspects of the activity can inspire new goalposts ... that are personally motivated, and therefore less about aesthetics or self-comparison with other dancers.

Body Image in Action: Consider starting a body gratitude practice. Reflect on or journal your responses to these questions: How did my body show up for me today? What did my body allow me to do today that I am thankful for? This practice can also be helpful to cope with body dissatisfaction and frustration that may occur during injury (e.g., I am thankful for my strong arms that help me get around on crutches. I am grateful for my eyes that can see the beautiful flowers my family sent me).

Challenging Narrow Beauty and Body Ideals

The beauty and body ideals that dancers (and the rest of us) are exposed to tend to be very narrow in terms of body size/shape, skin tone, hair, gender expression, etc. These restricted and constricting notions of what makes a person beautiful or one body type preferable over another harm everyone, but especially those who don't have the attributes that have been deemed ideal. Broadening your conceptualization of beauty supports more balanced body image.[11] Defining beauty broadly involves challenging socially constructed ideals so that all different body types, features, and appearances can be appreciated and perceived as beautiful.[8,17] It also means expanding your idea of beauty—in others and yourself—to go beyond just appearance to see beauty that emanates from within (e.g., from qualities such as kindness, confidence, joy).[8,17] When beauty is viewed in this way, you notice and appreciate the magnificence of human diversity and can counter comparison because each person is beautiful in their own unique way.[8]

Media, and social media in particular, plays a significant role in the perpetuation of unrealistic and harmful beauty and body standards.[11] Exposure to and internalization of these appearance ideals increases risk for and helps maintain body dissatisfaction and eating disorders/disordered eating.[17] Dancers need to be taught about the negative impact that media and the comparative process it generates can have on their body image and self-worth.[11] According to Spell, it's important to:

> [E]ncourage dancers to expand their view of a dancer's body. Utilizing social media as a benchmark for how a dancer's body and technique should look can sometimes lead to unrealistic and perfectionistic expectations. Diversifying one's feed and challenging one's bias can bring an additional layer of awareness and acceptance to one's own relationship with their body.

The more dancers are exposed to idealized and perfected images and messages, the more they believe these represent "real life,"[11] yet much of it isn't real at all. Dancers can learn how to critically evaluate and question what they read, hear, and see to help protect their body image and well-being. Encourage dancers to consider how images are created (e.g., are they digitally altered?), what message is being sent and its purpose (hint: it's often to sell something), and who might benefit from or be harmed by the message.[11] Dancers need to be empowered to challenge and reject content that propagates harmful ideals[8] and be mindful that their own content isn't inadvertently doing the same.[11] Reducing the amount of time spent on social media has also been shown to improve body image in vulnerable adolescents and young adults.[23]

Body Image in Action: Challenge yourself to seek out examples of non-appearance-based beauty in your daily life—someone savoring ice cream on a hot day, a moment of unrestrained laughter, an act of generosity that you witness.[17,20] Do a social media "detox"—unfollow accounts that negatively affect how you feel about yourself, experiment with taking a break from social media, or set limits on how much time you spend using it.

Loving Self-Care

Taking care of your body helps cultivate connection to and appreciation for it.[17] Dancers don't have to like the way their body looks to treat it well. In fact, showing care and compassion toward themselves may be especially important in moments when dancers feel negatively about their bodies because this reinforces through action that they are deserving of love and kindness no matter what their body looks/feels like. Notably, according to Catherine Cook-Cottone, "Mindful self-care and a positive body image may be reciprocal and self-perpetuating." In other words, as dancers practice taking care of themselves, they increase positive feelings toward themselves, and the better dancers feel about themselves, the more likely they are to engage in self-care.[17]

Loving self-care practices include[11,17]:

- Fueling your body consistently with foods that are nourishing and enjoyable
- Resting when you are tired
- Advocating for your needs and setting boundaries
- Going to healthcare appointments and taking needed medications/supplements
- Spending time with supportive people who model and encourage body acceptance and other healthy attitudes
- Filling your environment with things that bring you joy (e.g., artwork, inspirational messages, music you love)
- Doing things that feel comforting/soothing (e.g., getting a massage, wrapping yourself in a favorite blanket, spending time in nature)
- Using healthy coping tools for stress relief and to deal with difficult times
- Decreasing behaviors (e.g., dieting, punishing exercise, body checking, comparison) and exposure to people/media that contribute to negative feelings about your body or yourself

Body Image in Action: Are there any self-care practices listed above that you would like to commit to practicing or practicing more often? Are there any behaviors that you would benefit from reducing?

Practices to Promote Body Image Resiliency

Dancers will face situations and pressures that disrupt or threaten their relationship with their body such as hearing body comments, being told to change their body weight/shape/size, seeing a "bad" photo of themselves, injury, and many others. Although body image threats may be inevitable, the negative impact (or extent of that impact) on dancers' body image doesn't have to be. Enter body image resiliency. As described in a paper by Richardson and Waite, "The resiliency process is the experience of being disrupted by change, opportunities, adversity, stressors or challenges and, after some disorder, accessing personal gifts and strengths to grow stronger through the disruption." And resilience is "a self-righting force within everyone."[24]

Dancers can have negative body thoughts, feelings, and experiences and still have an overall positive body image. When body image disruptions occur, dancers have a choice in the outcome, and how they respond is key. That is not to say that harm from body shaming and other body image injuries can be completely undone. As discussed previously, the impacts from these experiences can last a lifetime. However, dancers can learn strategies to help them recover from body image threats and to bring some healing to existing body image wounds. At the same time, those who train and care for dancers must prioritize decreasing forces that contribute to negative body image in dancers because there is a limit to how resilient one can be in the face of multiple body image assaults. Below are a few additional practices that can help dancers build more resilient body image.

Learning from Discomfort

When negative body-related thoughts and feelings arise, it's beneficial for dancers to get curious about what's behind them to inform how they choose to respond. Sometimes feeling distress in or about the body doesn't actually have much to do with the body. Negative body thoughts and feelings can be a warning light indicating an unmet need (e.g., the need for rest, comfort, connection, or to feel valued). Or focusing on "fixing" your body might be serving as a coping mechanism or distraction from uncomfortable emotions.

It's also helpful to consider what contributes to the negative thoughts/ feelings, which provides insight on body protective changes to make. For example, if a dancer has more critical thoughts about their body when they are around certain people who engage in disparaging body talk, they might decide to speak out against body talk or limit time spent with these people. Like most types of healing, body image healing won't be linear, but each body image disruption offers an opportunity to learn and respond in a way that strengthens the resiliency muscle.

Reframing Negative Body Image Thoughts and Feelings

A dancer hears a peer get praised in class for losing weight. In reaction to this body image threat, the dancer may think, "My teacher doesn't like me because I'm too big." The dancer might feel sad, embarrassed, or angry at their body and decide to go on a restrictive diet. A more adaptive response would be to check for thought distortions or assumptions and reframe or counter them in a way that protects body image. This dancer might say to themselves: "Just because my teacher is praising another dancer doesn't mean they don't like me" or "I have my own unique gifts as a dancer."

The above dancer's thought was an assumption, not a fact. What if a dancer's thoughts and feelings are based on something they are explicitly told? For instance, a dancer is told they need to lose weight to fit into the costume for an upcoming performance. Or a dancer is told they are going to be taken out of a piece because of how their body looks. Thoughts like, "I won't get to dance this role if I don't lose weight" or "My director doesn't like how my body looks" are hard to refute. These examples illustrate the challenges to developing and maintaining positive (or neutral) body image in the dance world. Nevertheless, dancers can learn to cope with these body image threats in a way that hopefully lessens their negative impact. "What would you say to a friend?" is a helpful prompt to encourage responding to painful and difficult situations with the same kindness you would show to a loved one. Bringing in core values can also be useful. These dancers might say to themselves, "Body pressures in the dance world are so hard to deal with and I don't have to harm myself to meet unrealistic ideals" or "Costumes are meant to be altered to fit dancers, not dancers altered to fit costumes." Note: this is not easy to do!

Riding the Wave

No matter how much work a dancer has done on improving their body image, experiencing painful feelings in the face of body image threats such as the body shaming examples above is understandable and expected. Trying to deny, minimize, or disregard these emotions or judging them leads to more suffering.[2] On the other hand, making space for and accepting difficult feelings can help dancers cope in a way that supports body image healing.[11] In these moments, it may be useful to remember that, like an ocean wave, the intensity of painful emotions will recede. If possible, working with a therapist to learn distress tolerance skills can also be beneficial for dancers. As dancers practice riding the waves of their difficult feelings—going with them instead of fighting against them—they will return to calmer waters and see that they are strong enough to get through adversity.

Bouncing Back

Responding to body image threats in a self-protecting and caring (rather than self-harming) manner helps dancers bounce back from these negative experiences in a way that improves their relationship with their body (rather than degrading it). This means speaking to themselves with compassion and understanding and treating themselves with kindness by engaging in loving self-care.[11] Seeking professional help (e.g., from a psychotherapist, dietitian) can be of great benefit because trying to nourish balanced body image amidst the pressures and expectations of the dance world is no easy feat. In addition, having social and emotional support from friends and family plays an important role in body image satisfaction.[25] When dancers have people in their life who make them feel accepted as they are and for who they are, it can be a powerful force in nurturing positive (or neutral) body image.[11] This brings us back full circle to the need for a dance community and environment that will support dancers on their journey to developing more balanced and resilient body image.

Main Pointes

- A dancer's body image affects their physical and mental health, well-being, and performance.
- Internal and external factors influence the way dancers see themselves, what they think and how they feel about their body, how connected they are to their body, and how they behave toward it.
- Increasing connection to and aligning with core values can help dancers improve their body image.
- Practices such as body acceptance, body appreciation, challenging narrow beauty and body ideals, and attuned self-care can help dancers build more balanced body image.
- Dancers can have negative body thoughts, feelings, and experiences and still have an overall positive (or neutral) body image—how they respond to body image threats is key.

- Dancers can build body image resiliency by using body image disruptions as learning opportunities, reframing/countering negative thoughts, riding the wave of difficult emotions, and responding with care and compassion.
- Dancers need a community and environment that supports them in developing and practicing more balanced and resilient body image.

Notes

In your role/relationship with dancers, in what ways might you encourage body appreciation, acceptance, and/or attunement?

Did any of the concepts and practices discussed in this chapter resonate with you personally? Are there any steps that you'd like to take to improve your own body image?

Endnotes

* Body neutrality (having a neutral attitude toward the body, neither loving it nor hating it) is characterized by several elements covered in this chapter (e.g., functionality appreciation, respecting and caring for the body regardless of appearance, not defining self-worth by appearance).[26]
† This may be different for transgender individuals for whom changing their body to be more congruent with their gender identity may improve body acceptance.[11]

References

1. Radell SA, International Association for Dance Medicine & Science (IADMS). Mirrors in the dance class: Help or hindrance. Published online 2019. Accessed July 17, 2023. https://iadms.org/media/5781/iadms-resource-paper-mirrors-in-the-dance-class.pdf
2. Cash T. *The Body Image Workbook: An Eight-Step Program for Learning to Like Your Looks.* Second ed. New Harbinger Publications; 2008:232.
3. Grogan S. *Body Image: Understanding Body Dissatisfaction in Men, Women, and Children.* 4th ed. Routledge; 2021:266. doi:10.4324/9781003100041
4. Piran N. Embodied possibilities and disruptions: The emergence of the experience of embodiment construct from qualitative studies with girls and women. *Body Image.* 2016;18:43–60. doi:10.1016/j.bodyim.2016.04.007
5. Davison KK, Markey CN, Birch LL. Etiology of body dissatisfaction and weight concerns among 5-year-old girls. *Appetite.* 2000;35(2):143–151. doi:10.1006/appe.2000.0349
6. Hosseini SA, Padhy RK. Body image distortion. In: *StatPearls.* StatPearls Publishing; 2023.
7. Arcelus J, Witcomb GL, Mitchell A. Prevalence of eating disorders amongst dancers: A systemic review and meta-analysis. *Eur Eat Disord Rev.* 2014;22(2):92–101. doi:10.1002/erv.2271
8. Tylka TL, Wood-Barcalow NL. What is and what is not positive body image? Conceptual foundations and construct definition. *Body Image.* 2015;14:118–129. doi:10.1016/j.bodyim.2015.04.001

9. Mustillo SA, Hendrix KL, Schafer MH. Trajectories of body mass and self-concept in black and white girls: The lingering effects of stigma. *J Health Soc Behav*. 2012;53(1):2–16. doi:10.1177/0022146511419205

10. Doria N, Numer M. Dancing in a culture of disordered eating: A feminist poststructural analysis of body and body image among young girls in the world of dance. *PLoS ONE*. 2022;17(1):e0247651. doi:10.1371/journal.pone.0247651

11. Wood-Barcalow N, Tylka T, Judge C. *Positive Body Image Workbook: A Clinical and Self-Improvement Guide*. Cambridge University Press; 2021:372.

12. Kinavey H, Sturtevant D. *Reclaiming Body Trust: A Path to Healing & Liberation*. TarcherPerigee; 2022:320.

13. Tribole E, Resch E. *Intuitive Eating, 4th Edition: A Revolutionary Anti-Diet Approach*. 2nd ed. St. Martin's Essentials; 2020:392.

14. Boswell JF, Anderson LM, Oswald JM, Reilly EE, Gorrell S, Anderson DA. A preliminary naturalistic clinical case series study of the feasibility and impact of interoceptive exposure for eating disorders. *Behav Res Ther*. 2019;117:54–64. doi:10.1016/j.brat.2019.02.004

15. Badoud D, Tsakiris M. From the body's viscera to the body's image: Is there a link between interoception and body image concerns? *Neurosci Biobehav Rev*. 2017;77:237–246. doi:10.1016/j.neubiorev.2017.03.017

16. Quadt L, Critchley HD, Garfinkel SN. The neurobiology of interoception in health and disease. *Ann N Y Acad Sci*. 2018;1428(1):112–128. doi:10.1111/nyas.13915

17. Cook-Cottone CP. Incorporating positive body image into the treatment of eating disorders: A model for attunement and mindful self-care. *Body Image*. 2015;14:158–167. doi:10.1016/j.bodyim.2015.03.004

18. Mindful Staff. Jon Kabat-Zinn: Defining mindfulness. January 11, 2017. Accessed July 28, 2023. https://www.mindful.org/jon-kabat-zinn-defining-mindfulness/

19. Fischer D, Messner M, Pollatos O. Improvement of interoceptive processes after an 8-week body scan intervention. *Front Hum Neurosci*. 2017;11:452. doi:10.3389/fnhum.2017.00452

20. Cook-Cottone C. *Embodiment and the Treatment of Eating Disorders: The Body as a Resource in Recovery*. 1st ed. W. W. Norton; 2020:384.

21. Piran N. Taking Space: Perils, Pleasures, and Privilege. Presented at: iaedp Virtual Symposium; 2023.

22. Braun TD, Park CL, Gorin A. Self-compassion, body image, and disordered eating: A review of the literature. *Body Image*. 2016;17:117–131. doi:10.1016/j.bodyim.2016.03.003

23. Thai H, Davis CG, Mahboob W, Perry S, Adams A, Goldfield GS. Reducing social media use improves appearance and weight esteem in youth with emotional distress. *Psychol Pop Media*. February 27, 2023. doi:10.1037/ppm0000460

24. Richardson GE, Waite PJ. Mental health promotion through resilience and resiliency education. *Int J Emerg Ment Health*. 2002;4(1):65–75.

25. Merianos A, King K, Vidourek R. Does perceived social support play a role in body image satisfaction among college students? *J Behav Health*. 2012;1(3):178–184. doi:10.5455/jbh.20120501101051

26. Pellizzer ML, Wade TD. Developing a definition of body neutrality and strategies for an intervention. *Body Image*. 2023;46:434–442. doi:10.1016/j.bodyim.2023.07.006

9 Whole Dancer Health

Dancers are developing people first and foremost. We need to nurture their emotional, physical, and psychological needs simultaneously during training instead of trying to keep these aspects of development separate.

~Josh Spell, LICSW, consulting therapist for Pacific Northwest Ballet School and Company

Nurturing and supporting dancers' health requires considering the whole dancer—their mind, body, and spirit. Prior chapters covered important areas of concern for dancers' health including dieting, under-fueling, eating disorders/disordered eating, injury, and body image. This chapter touches on a few additional aspects, focusing on those that impact how dancers nourish and care for themselves and their relationship with food and their body. Figure 9.1 illustrates various facets of dancer health addressed in this book, which are interrelated and directly and indirectly influence each other.

Sleep

Getting enough good quality sleep is critical for dancers' physical and mental health and performance. Poor sleep can negatively impact muscle strength, reaction time, learning, memory, creativity, mood, immune function, and increase injury risk.[1,2] Nutrition and mental health have reciprocal relationships with sleep.[1] For example, not eating enough can affect sleep[3] and not sleeping enough can affect eating.[4,5] Insufficient sleep can exacerbate symptoms of depression and anxiety, and depression and anxiety may impair sleep.[1,6]

Although sleep needs can be variable, general recommendations based on age are:

* **Adults**: 7 or more hours/night[7]
* **Teenagers** (13–18 years old): 8–10 hours/night[8]
* **School-age children** (6–12 years old): 9–12 hours/night[8]

DOI: 10.4324/9781003366171-12

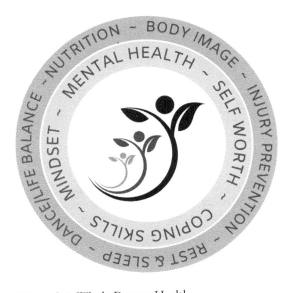

Figure 9.1 Whole Dancer Health.
Created by the author (image credit © Marsono from UPgraphic via Canva.com).

Dancers may need more sleep than this to help them recover from the mental and physical stresses of training.[9,10] The higher a dancer's training load and the greater stress they are under, the more crucial it is to get enough sleep.[9,11] Researcher Cheri Mah, an expert on sleep and performance in athletes, recommends that adult elite athletes get 8–10 or more hours of sleep every night.[12] It has also been suggested that athletes who train 4–6 hours a day may benefit from 10–12 hours of sleep per night.[13] However, there are individual differences in the amount of sleep needed for optimal health and performance.[7] The goal is for dancers to sleep for the amount of time that they require to feel awake and alert throughout the day.[9]

Unfortunately, poor sleep is common in dancers.[14,15] The same factors that increase the importance of sleep (i.e., high training load and stress) can also negatively impact it.[9,10] In addition, dancers' schedules (e.g., evening performances and early morning class), touring, and non-ideal sleep habits (e.g., scrolling on social media in bed) can interfere with obtaining sufficient sleep.[10] The good news is that short naps of around 30 minutes can help sleep-deprived dancers, though it's best not to nap too late in the day so nighttime sleep is not affected.[9] Table 9.1 provides other strategies to improve sleep quality and quantity.

Table 9.1 Tips to Improve Sleep

Try to keep a consistent sleep schedule (i.e., go to bed and wake up at the same time each day).
Turn off the television and stop using phones, tablets, and other electronic devices at least one hour before bed.
Avoid caffeine and alcohol too close to bedtime.
Implement a relaxing pre-sleep routine—take a warm bath, read a book, journal, or do a guided meditation.
Make your bedroom dark, cool, and quiet to support uninterrupted sleep. If needed, consider using a sleep mask, earplugs, and/or a white noise machine.

Adapted from Ordóñez et al.,[2] Bird,[9] and National Sleep Foundation.[16]

Wakeful Rest

In addition to sleep, dancers need other forms of downtime and rest to help their body repair and recover, to give their mind the break it needs to feel restored, and to prevent overtraining and burnout.* For wakeful rest to be rejuvenating, dancers should do things that don't require much physical or intellectual effort and provide a break from thinking about dance (e.g., reading, watching television or a movie, doing a non-physically active hobby, or spending time with friends in a relaxed setting).[17]

Busy dance schedules make it challenging to find time to rest as limited time off may need to be spent taking care of errands, chores, and other to-dos. The busier dancers are, the more important it is to prioritize rest during the breaks they have within each day, on days off, and in their off-season. For example, although dancers might want to squeeze in extra practice or conditioning when they have a break between rehearsals, they will likely benefit more from using this time to sit and eat a meal or snack, put their feet up and relax, or even take a short nap. Dancers' bodies are usually screaming for rest by the end of a season/semester, yet they may struggle to honor this need because of concern that they will get out of shape or lose valuable time when they "should" be improving their technique, or because they have a hard time giving themselves permission to rest. Dancers may think of rest as "doing nothing" and feel guilty or lazy if they "waste time" not being productive. Not only is rest productive, but dancers also need to challenge the idea that they must be productive at all times. Dancers may need to be taught or reminded that—for the sake of their physical and mental health, performance, and longevity as a dancer—sometimes less is more!

Managing Perfectionism

Perfectionism is a multidimensional personality trait that involves setting excessively high personal standards of performance as well as the tendency for overly critical self-evaluation.[18,19] Some aspects of perfectionism, such as striving for high standards and being driven and determined, are not necessarily problematic and may be fundamental to dancers' success.[20] However, other characteristics of perfectionism such as worrying about mistakes, self-doubt, self-criticism, and feeling that what you do is never good enough can be harmful to dancers' performance and health.[20] Studies have found that perfectionism is associated with eating disorder development, anxiety, injury, and burnout.[20]

Some research studies refer to a type of perfectionism that is "healthy," positive, or adaptive where an individual has high personal standards but isn't overly distressed or self-critical when they don't achieve these standards.[21-23] Others disagree with this conceptualization and say that possessing the positive part of perfectionism without the negative side is better described as striving for excellence, not perfectionism.[20,24] It is beyond the scope of this chapter to cover the varying models and proposed dimensions of perfectionism. However, although perfectionism may include both adaptive and maladaptive features with the degree of each varying among individuals,[19] it's rare to be a perfectionist and not experience some of the negative attributes.[20] Given how common perfectionistic tendencies are among dancers,[25,26] it's important to help them learn how to better manage the detrimental aspects.

Perfectionism is associated with dichotomous (aka black-and-white) thinking.[21] I often see this type of thinking manifest in and affect dancers' relationship with food and exercise. For example, they view their eating as either good or bad, and if they eat a "bad" or off-limits food, they feel their day is ruined. They might think that if a meal isn't perfect, it's not worth eating. Or if they don't run a certain number of miles, it doesn't count as exercise. Or they don't cook because they believe they are bad at it. It's helpful for dancers to learn how to challenge and reframe these distortions (e.g., All foods can fit. Food is meant to be nourishing and enjoyable—sometimes it's more of one than the other, and that's okay. Making mistakes is how you learn.).

Sasha Gorrell, Licensed Clinical Psychologist in the University of California, San Francisco Eating Disorders Program, finds it helpful "to encourage dancers to try some perspective taking. [For example], if you saw one of your friends never taking a day off, do you think that is sustainable?" She also says it's important to help dancers recognize the difference between what they need to do or give up to dance well, and what constitutes maladaptive perfectionism. Spell helps dancers learn about the function perfectionism serves for them, which

> often reveals an element of attempting to avoid failure or mediocrity (fear of failure, fear of making a mistake, fear of being seen as incompetent) through relentless self-criticism. Identifying the self-critic and some of the unsustainable outcomes the critic is trying to achieve can bring some awareness to the false sense of control that perfectionism brings.

There may also be other needs, such as the need to feel accepted, that drive perfectionistic behavior and that are important to address.[24] Notably, Gorrell, Spell, and Philippa Ziegenhardt, qualified Counsellor and the former School Counsellor for The Australian Ballet School, all highlight the importance of self-compassion to help dancers counter self-criticism and manage the other harmful aspects of perfectionism.

Matters of the Mind

You can't control all the thoughts that pop into your mind, but you do have a say in how and how much they affect you. Thoughts are influenced by environment, lived experience, and what you believe about yourself and the world (i.e., core beliefs); and your thoughts in turn influence your feelings, sensations in your body, and your behaviors.[27] Many thoughts are automatic. Some are fleeting and have little or no emotional impact while others—especially repetitive negative thoughts and judgments about yourself, others, or the future—can cause significant distress.[27]

As discussed in Chapter 8, dancers may have negative thoughts and feelings that make sense given the situation, and they can learn to respond with self-compassion and self-care. Other times, negative thoughts and feelings are related to unhelpful thinking patterns (aka "thinking traps" or cognitive distortions).[27] Figure 9.2[†] shows how two different dancers react to not getting cast in a piece. Although Jordan understandably feels disappointed, their response is adaptive and supportive of their physical and mental health and dance goals. Jamie's thoughts illustrate cognitive distortions (e.g., reaching a conclusion without specific evidence to support it)[28] and their effect.

Comparison is a thinking trap that is common among dancers. Psychotherapist and Certified Eating Disorder Specialist Dawn Smith-Theodore works with dancers "on how they can focus on themself and not compare to other dancers, whether it be their body, technique, or parts that they get." According to Ziegenhardt, "Learning to recognize and dispute unhelpful thinking can empower dancers, even from a young age, to think more realistically." For dancers who are "stuck in a rut of thinking," Gorrell suggests

> [holding] open the door to a less myopic view of things. [For example], this might be fine right now, but if you keep this attitude, how will next season look? Is this way of thinking going to be sustainable if we checked back in on you in five years?

It's beneficial for dancers to be reminded of what they can control (e.g., fueling before an audition) and what they can't (e.g., getting a part) to counter distorted thoughts and self-defeating reactions and coping mechanisms.

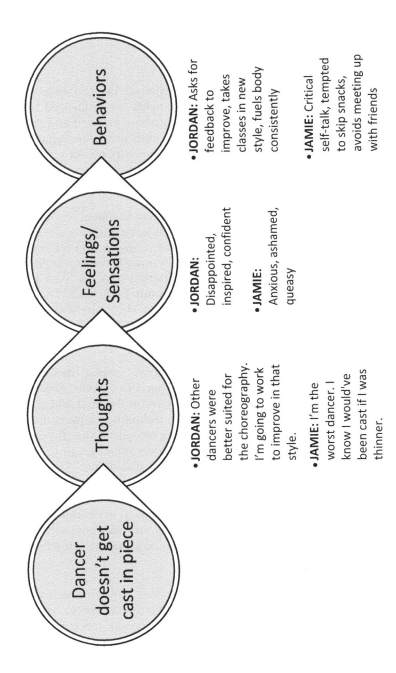

Figure 9.2 Two Reactions to the Same Event.

Spell teaches dancers about Circles of Control to help "bring [them] from the reactive into the proactive." He reminds dancers about "what is in their purview of control regardless of how large or small (picking out a leotard for class, ... what warm up exercises or stretches to engage in before class, what intention to set before class)." Spell adds, "Reminding dancers that other people or casting are not in their control can help separate feelings of powerlessness and instead promote empowerment."

In addition, Ziegenhardt says it's helpful for dancers to learn about how the brain works and how it tries to protect us. This understanding can help dancers be compassionate toward themselves as they bring awareness to unhelpful thinking patterns that might be negatively impacting their thoughts, feelings, and behaviors. Then they can work to reframe or redirect thoughts in a way that supports their physical and mental health, performance, and a healthy relationship with food and their body.

Returning to Figure 9.2, Jordan's response illustrates a growth mindset—they viewed the disappointment of not getting cast as a chance to learn and improve. According to researcher and psychologist Carol Dweck,[29] individuals who have a growth mindset think of their talent and ability as something they can develop with effort, practice, and feedback. On the other hand, someone with a fixed mindset believes their ability is innate—they only have a certain amount and there's not much they can do about it. Dancers with a growth mindset focus on learning and embrace challenges, which means doing things they might not feel good at. Dancers with a fixed mindset may give up when faced with a setback or turn down opportunities that could lead to growth because they are afraid to expose perceived weaknesses.[29]

Studies have shown that a growth mindset is associated with more adaptive coping and better mental health and performance.[29-32] The good news is that because mindsets are beliefs, they can be changed.[29] According to Ziegenhardt, self-compassion is the best in-road to help dancers develop more of a growth mindset: "Without it, it's just a theory and pressure and [dancers] get upset with themselves for not having the 'right' mindset, which adds another layer of emotion to deal with when they are already being hard on themselves."

Dance/Life Balance

Being a dancer is an identity, but it's not the only thing that defines who a dancer is. The demands and pressures of the dance world can make it challenging to find time and mental space for much else. But dedication to dance should not come at the expense of dancers' physical, emotional, and social needs, or self-development.[33,34] Over-identification as a dancer may increase the risk of poor body image and burnout.[35,36] In addition, if a dancer's sense of self-worth and value disproportionately come from dance and the feedback they get in this realm, it can make dealing with disruptions in their ability to participate (e.g., due to injury, retirement, not getting selected for a part or program) more difficult and destabilizing.[36,37]

Dance can provide a great deal for dancers—a creative and emotional outlet, confidence, fulfillment, and much more—but it's not healthy if it's the be-all and end-all of their existence.[20] Even for dancers who need to spend most of their time training and performing, it's important to nourish an identity separate from dance. Dancers need to be encouraged to explore non-dance interests, socialize with non-dance friends, and make time for play. Gorrell offers this advice:

> I think developing and cultivating social support that lies outside of the dance world can be particularly promoting of wellbeing. Of course, dance peers are your family, but it's helpful to have other close confidantes outside of that group to provide a more objective and unbiased sounding board.

In addition, by expanding their sense of identity through life experiences, dancers will be more resilient and have more to offer as artists.[20] Finding dance/life balance is important for dancers' health, quality of life, and their dancing.

Coping Tools

When interviewing dance psychotherapists for this book, I asked, "What skills/tools/behaviors do you think dancers need to help them cope with the pressures of the dance world and to support their health and well-being?" A compiled list of beneficial coping strategies for dancers based on their responses is shown in Table 9.2. Additional guidance to help dancers cope with injury and body image threats was provided in Chapters 7 and 8, respectively.

Table 9.2 Coping Skills and Strategies for Dancers

Relaxation techniques (e.g., breathing exercises, progressive muscle relaxation)[38]	Mindfulness
Self-compassion	Assertive communication
Distress tolerance	Critical thinking
Mental imagery	Filtering feedback
Goal setting	Psychological flexibility
Boundary setting	Grounding/centering practices (e.g., meditation)
Positive self-talk[39]	Self-reflection practices (e.g., journaling)[38]

Adapted from interviews with Sasha Gorrell, Josh Spell, and Philippa Ziegenhardt with additional sources as indicated.

How You Can Help

This chapter began with a quote from a dance psychotherapist and ends with another, this time from Sasha Gorrell:

> As much as a performance focus is appropriate in the dance world, I would like to see a paradigm shift to a "whole health" focus. ... In the long term, this shift would also promote performance. ... I wish the industry would play more of a long game, helping the dancers to cultivate a more well-rounded sense of their identity both within and outside dance, and to learn how to take care of themselves and develop self-care and psychological skills that will serve them life-long.

You can encourage and help dancers to cultivate the attitudes and practices discussed in this chapter by modeling getting adequate sleep and rest, having realistic expectations for yourself, finding work/life balance, using healthy coping tools, etc. Here are a few additional suggestions for how you can support dancers:

- Dancers' need for rest should be accounted for when planning schedules. For dance educators/artistic staff/leadership, this means considering the intensity and volume of training/performing within daily schedules as well as throughout the season/semester (e.g., building in lighter days before an intense performance period).[40] For parents, this might mean planning family time with your busy dancer that is relaxing rather than physically active.
- Parents/caregivers—set limits on when and where screentime is allowed (e.g., not right before or in bed) and help your dancer set and stick to a regular bedtime so they can meet their sleep needs.
- Help dancers set challenging, realistic, and specific goals that are within their control (i.e., that consider their personal ability).[20]
- Rather than complimenting natural talent, praise dancers' effort, progress, and how they approach challenges.[29]
- Explicitly state that you are not looking for perfection.[20]
- Spell offers this advice for those who train and care for dancers: "normalize making mistakes and promote more kind, collaborative, and nurturing feedback." Similarly, for teachers and parents, Ziegenhardt recommends "[s]etting realistic expectations and allowing enough time and experimentation to grow."

Main Pointes

- Adequate sleep is critical for dancers' health and performance. The higher their training load and the greater stress they are under, the more crucial it is to get enough sleep.

- Dancers also need wakeful rest to help their body repair and recover, give their mind the break it needs to feel restored, and prevent overtraining and burnout.
- Self-compassion is key to helping dancers manage harmful aspects of perfectionism, identify and reframe unhelpful thinking patterns, and nurture a growth mindset.
- Dance/life balance is important for dancers' health, quality of life, and their dancing.

Notes

Do you struggle personally with any of the areas discussed in this chapter (e.g., not getting enough sleep/rest, managing perfectionism, etc.)? If so, how do you think this might impact your work or relationship with dancers?

Endnotes

* Overtraining happens when there is an imbalance between stress (from training and life) and recovery (i.e., too much stress and not enough regeneration)[11] leading to impaired performance and symptoms such as fatigue, mood changes, loss of appetite, and increased illnesses and injury.[41,42] Burnout describes a state of emotional and physical exhaustion that shares many of the symptoms of overtraining plus a loss of interest, motivation, and enjoyment in dance.[41,42]
† Thoughts, feelings, and behaviors have a more interrelated relationship than depicted in Figure 9.2 (e.g., thoughts influence feelings/sensations and vice versa; behaviors can lead to consequences that reinforce thoughts; etc.).[27]

References

1. Charest J, Grandner MA. Sleep and athletic performance: Impacts on physical performance, mental performance, injury risk and recovery, and mental health. *Sleep Med Clin.* 2020;15(1):41–57. doi:10.1016/j.jsmc.2019.11.005
2. Ordóñez FM, Sanchez-Oliver AJ, Carrera-Bastos P, Guillén LS, Domínguez R. Sleep improvement in athletes: Use of nutritional supplements. *Arch Med Deporte.* 2017;34:93–99.
3. Gillbanks L, Mountjoy M, Filbay SR. Lightweight rowers' perspectives of living with Relative Energy Deficiency in Sport (RED-S). *PLoS ONE.* 2022;17(3):e0265268. doi:10.1371/journal.pone.0265268
4. Halson SL. Sleep in elite athletes and nutritional interventions to enhance sleep. *Sports Med.* 2014;44 Suppl 1(1):S13–23. doi:10.1007/s40279-014-0147-0
5. Chaput J-P, Dutil C. Lack of sleep as a contributor to obesity in adolescents: Impacts on eating and activity behaviors. *Int J Behav Nutr Phys Act.* 2016;13(1):103. doi:10.1186/s12966-016-0428-0
6. Franzen PL, Buysse DJ. Sleep disturbances and depression: Risk relationships for subsequent depression and therapeutic implications. *Dialogues Clin Neurosci.* 2008;10(4):473–481. doi:10.31887/DCNS.2008.10.4/plfranzen
7. Watson NF, Badr MS, Belenky G, et al. Recommended amount of sleep for a healthy adult: A joint consensus statement of the American Academy of Sleep

Medicine and sleep research society. *Sleep*. 2015;38(6):843–844. doi:10.5665/sleep.4716

8. Paruthi S, Brooks LJ, D'Ambrosio C, et al. Recommended amount of sleep for pediatric populations: A consensus statement of the American Academy of Sleep Medicine. *J Clin Sleep Med*. 2016;12(6):785–786. doi:10.5664/jcsm.5866

9. Bird S. Sleep, recovery, and athletic performance: A brief review and recommendations. *Strength Cond J*. 2013;35:43–47.

10. Walsh NP, Halson SL, Sargent C, et al. Sleep and the athlete: Narrative review and 2021 expert consensus recommendations. *Br J Sports Med*. November 3, 2020. doi:10.1136/bjsports-2020-102025

11. Kellmann M. Underrecovery and overtraining: Different concepts – Similar impact? *Olympic Coach*. 2003;15(3):4–7.

12. Rosenberg A. How to sleep like a pro (Athlete). UCSF Clinical & Translational Science Institute. February 18, 2016. Accessed August 19, 2023. https://ctsi.ucsf.edu/news/how-sleep-pro-athlete

13. Scott WA. Maximizing performance and the prevention of injuries in competitive athletes. *Curr Sports Med Rep*. 2002;1(3):184–190. doi:10.1249/00149619-200206000-00010

14. Michaels C, Holman A, Teramoto M, Bellendir T, Krautgasser-Tolman S, Willick SE. Descriptive analysis of mental and physical wellness in collegiate dancers. *J Dance Med Sci*. 2023;27(3):173-179. doi:10.1177/1089313X231178091

15. Arbinaga F. Self-reported perceptions of sleep quality and resilience among dance students. *Percept Mot Skills*. 2018;125(2):351–368. doi:10.1177/0031512518757352

16. National Sleep Foundation. Healthy sleep starts before you hit the sheets. March 13, 2022. Accessed August 19, 2023. https://www.thensf.org/healthy-sleep-starts-before-you-hit-the-sheets/

17. Eccles DW, Kazmier AW. The psychology of rest in athletes: An empirical study and initial model. *Psychol Sport Exerc*. 2019;44:90–98. doi:10.1016/j.psychsport.2019.05.007

18. Frost RO, Marten P, Lahart C, Rosenblate R. The dimensions of perfectionism. *Cognit Ther Res*. 1990;14(5):449–468. doi:10.1007/BF01172967

19. Nordin-Bates SM, Raedeke TD, Madigan DJ. Perfectionism, burnout, and motivation in dance: A replication and test of the 2×2 model of perfectionism. *J Dance Med Sci*. 2017;21(3):115–122. doi:10.12678/1089-313X.21.3.115

20. Nordin-Bates S, International Association for Dance Medicine & Science. Perfectionism. Published online 2014. Accessed August 20, 2023. https://iadms.org/media/5910/iadms-resource-paper-perfectionism.pdf

21. Egan SJ, Piek JP, Dyck MJ, Rees CS. The role of dichotomous thinking and rigidity in perfectionism. *Behav Res Ther*. 2007;45(8):1813–1822. doi:10.1016/j.brat.2007.02.002

22. Bieling PJ, Israeli AL, Antony MM. Is perfectionism good, bad, or both? Examining models of the perfectionism construct. *Pers Individ Dif*. 2004;36(6):1373–1385. doi:10.1016/S0191-8869(03)00235-6

23. Rice KG, Bair CJ, Castro JR, Cohen BN, Hood CA. Meanings of perfectionism: A quantitative and qualitative analysis. *J Cogn Psychother*. 2003;17(1):39–58. doi:10.1891/jcop.17.1.39.58266

24. Benson E. The many faces of perfectionism. American Psychological Association. November 2003. Accessed August 20, 2023. https://www.apa.org/monitor/nov03/manyfaces

25. Nordin-Bates SM, Cumming J, Aways D, Sharp L. Imagining yourself dancing to perfection? Correlates of perfectionism among ballet and contemporary dancers. *J Clin Sport Psychol.* 2011;5(1):58–76. doi:10.1123/jcsp.5.1.58

26. Pentith R, Moss SL, Lamb K, Edwards C. Perfectionism among young female competitive Irish dancers – Prevalence and relationship with injury responses. *J Dance Med Sci.* 2021;25(2):152–158. doi:10.12678/1089-313X.061521k

27. Josefowitz N, Myran D. *CBT Made Simple: A Clinician's Guide to Practicing Cognitive Behavioral Therapy.* New Harbinger Publications; 2017:256.

28. Yurica CL, DiTomasso RA. Cognitive Distortions. In: Freeman A, Felgoise SH, Nezu CM, Nezu AM, Reinecke MA, eds. *Encyclopedia of Cognitive Behavior Therapy.* Springer; 2005:117–122. doi:10.1007/0-306-48581-8_36

29. Dweck CS. Mindsets: Developing talent through a growth mindset. *Olympic Coach.* 2009;21(1):4–7.

30. Burnette JL, Knouse LE, Vavra DT, O'Boyle E, Brooks MA. Growth mindsets and psychological distress: A meta-analysis. *Clin Psychol Rev.* 2020;77:101816. doi:10.1016/j.cpr.2020.101816

31. McNeil DG, Phillips WJ, Scoggin SA. Examining the importance of athletic mindset profiles for level of sport performance and coping. *Int J Sport Exerc Psychol.* February 22, 2023:1–17. doi:10.1080/1612197X.2023.2180073

32. Tao W, Zhao D, Yue H, et al. The influence of growth mindset on the mental health and life events of college students. *Front Psychol.* 2022;13:821206. doi:10.3389/fpsyg.2022.821206

33. Dwarika MS, Haraldsen HM. Mental health in dance: A scoping review. *Front Psychol.* 2023;14:1090645. doi:10.3389/fpsyg.2023.1090645

34. van Staden A, Myburgh CPH, Poggenpoel M. A psycho-educational model to enhance the self-development and mental health of classical dancers. *J Dance Med Sci.* 2009;13(1):20–28.

35. Langdon SW, Petracca G. Tiny dancer: Body image and dancer identity in female modern dancers. *Body Image.* 2010;7(4):360–363. doi:10.1016/j.bodyim.2010.06.005

36. Mainwaring L. Identity matters. July 14, 2019. Accessed August 24, 2023. https://iadms.org/resources/blog/posts/2019/july/identity-matters/

37. Darpinian S, Sterling W, Aggarwal S. *Raising Body Positive Teens: A Parent's Guide to Diet-Free Living, Exercise, and Body Image.* Jessica Kingsley Publishers; 2022:224.

38. Grove JR, Main LC, Sharp L. Stressors, recovery processes, and manifestations of training distress in dance. *J Dance Med Sci.* 2013;17(2):70–78. doi:10.12678/1089-313x.17.2.70

39. Noh Y-E, Morris T, Andersen MB. Psychological intervention programs for reduction of injury in ballet dancers. *Res Sports Med.* 2007;15(1):13–32. doi:10.1080/15438620600987064

40. Wyon M. Preparing to perform: Periodization and dance. *J Dance Med Sci.* 2010;14(2):67–72.

41. Lemyre P-N, Roberts GC, Stray-Gundersen J. Motivation, overtraining, and burnout: Can self-determined motivation predict overtraining and burnout in elite athletes? *Eur J Sport Sci.* 2007;7(2):115–126. doi:10.1080/17461390701302607

42. Kinucan P, Kravitz L. Overtraining: Undermining success? *ACSMs Health Fit J.* 2007;11(4):8–12. doi:10.1249/01.FIT.0000281225.23643.05

Epilogue

We are at a critical crossroads in the dance world. On one side, there are those who understand that change is needed to make dance environments healthier and safer for dancers and who are ready to embrace this change. On the other side, there are some who continue holding on to the old ways of doing things and push back against progress.

The pull to stay with tradition and the familiar is understandable. It can be hard to let go of deeply ingrained diet and dance culture beliefs. This book might be your first exposure to information that challenges ideas you've taken at face value. You may have sacrificed a lot buying into these beliefs. You may need time to process and to become more open to the idea that there could be another way. A better way.

The passing down of dance and its traditions from generation to generation is a beautiful aspect of this art form. It can be complicated to question the ways in which you were trained, especially if they were beneficial to you (e.g., if you were shamed into losing weight and rewarded with career advancement). Maybe you feel that the sacrifice was worth it or believe that this is just how the dance world needs to be because this is how it's always been. Or, though rare, perhaps you made it through relatively unscathed.

Meaningful change in the dance world will take our collective effort. It will require us to be courageous and view our past through a lens of new knowledge. It will require us to be willing to see and understand perspectives different from our own. We have the voices of dancers sharing their lived experiences to guide us and a good deal of research on the impact of practices, pressures, and expectations in dance that we can't afford to ignore. As Suvi Honkanen writes, "no art is good art if it leaves broken artists behind."[1]

Dance is an aesthetic art which means that focus on the body is necessary, and there are undeniable practical considerations that influence existing body preferences. But are we willing to accept the cost of the current narrow "ideals" that exist in much of the dance world? Does our field want to continue to demand "ideals" that are unattainable for most or require dancers to harm their physical and mental health to achieve? Or is there room to expand what we think a dancer's body is supposed to look like? Are we willing to do the work of challenging our biases to protect the humans without whom there is no art?

DOI: 10.4324/9781003366171-13

Change is possible and shifts are happening in the dance world. It's encouraging to see more diversity of body types, race/ethnicity, and gender starting to be represented. I am so grateful for the schools and companies that are committed to providing their dancers and staff with education and resources related to nutrition, mental health, and eating disorders. Yet there is much more to be done. Imagine what might shift if nurturing positive body image and a healthy relationship with food were part of every dance school's mission. What if all dance curriculum included teaching dancers how to care for themselves as humans and as dancers? Prioritizing dancers' health and well-being is necessary if we want them and the art form to thrive.

I hope this book has made you want to be a part of the change that is so needed in the dance world. And if you've already been working as an agent of change, I hope this book has given you motivation to continue the mission. Before we part, I invite you to consider if there is one new or additional step you can take toward the change you wish to see.

We have a choice to make at this fork in the road. The more of us who go down the new path toward a healthier and safer dance world, the more well-travelled it will become, and the less used and visible the former path will be. Soon the old way will no longer feel like a good option to take. Although this marks the end of this part of our time together, I hope it will not be the end of our shared journey to build a better dance world.

Reference

1. Honkanen S. As ballet looks toward its future, let's talk about its troubling emotional demands. *Pointe*. February 21, 2021. Accessed August 27, 2023. https://pointemagazine.com/ballet-and-emotional-demands/

Acknowledgments

I would not have been able to write this book without the love, encouragement, guidance, and help of many. Thank you to my brilliant and generous friend Jenna Hollenstein for pushing me to write this book and providing advice and support throughout the process (it might have taken me another ten years to start if not for your loving nudges). Thank you to my content readers—Sasha Gorrell, Fiona Sutherland, Jennifer M. Gómez, Stephanie Potreck, and Jenna—for your invaluable feedback and suggestions. I am so grateful for every colleague and friend who shared their expertise, checked in on me, and provided vital encouragement, cheerleading, advice, and support along the way including Dana Panepinto, Maya Menendez, Robin Millet, Justine Roth, Jasmine Challis, and Heidi Skolnik.

Thank you to Sasha Gorrell, Dawn Smith-Theodore, Josh Spell, Philippa Ziegenhardt, Julie Daugherty, Jessica Lassiter, Marissa Schaeffer, and Andrea Zujko for allowing me to interview you and share your expertise with the readers. I wish I had space to include more of your wise words! Thank you to Melissa Kirk for helping me through the book proposal process, Colleen Clemens for your editing (and word cutting) skills, and David Varley for believing in this book.

I owe great thanks to the researchers, writers, clinicians, and activists in the non-diet, eating disorder, and dance medicine spaces from whom I have learned so much and whose work forms the foundation upon which this book was built. To the dancers I interviewed, thank you for sharing your lived experiences which greatly enriched this book. To all my clients, thank you for giving me the privilege of being a part of your journey; entrusting me with your stories, struggles, and triumphs; and for being my greatest teachers.

I would not be me without dance and this book wouldn't exist without my life as a dancer. I am filled with gratitude for my dance teachers (too many to name) who taught me so much about dance, life, and myself. Thank you to Diana Byer for taking a chance on me and giving me an opportunity to live my dream and thank you to Cameron Gomez for keeping me dancing for the past decade.

Lastly, but most importantly, much love and gratitude for my family. Thank you to my mom for giving us the gift of the arts from a very young age. To my dad, thank you for modeling hard work and perseverance, which have guided my way in writing this book and throughout my life. Thank you to my brother Rajiv for your support and study access! And the biggest thank you to my husband Scott for your patience, encouragement, and support through this grueling and often all-consuming process—with your help, I made it across the finish line in time!

If I've forgotten anyone, please forgive me—you are appreciated.

Gracias. Shukriya. Thank you.

Appendix

The below resources offer additional information on topics discussed in this book. This list is not all-inclusive, nor does it represent a full endorsement of every piece of information included in each resource or provided by the organizations, especially for websites which frequently change/update content. However, I and many of my clients and colleagues have found these resources helpful and I hope you will too.

Books

The ABCs of Body-Positive Parenting (e-resource) by The Full Bloom Project

The Black Dancing Body: A Geography from Coon to Cool by Brenda Dixon Gottschild

Eating Disorders in Sport by Ron A. Thompson and Roberta Trattner Sherman

Fat Talk: Parenting in the Age of Diet Culture by Virginia Sole-Smith

Fearing the Black Body: The Racial Origins of Fat Phobia by Sabrina Strings

How to Nourish Your Child Through an Eating Disorder: A Simple, Plate-by-Plate Approach® to Rebuilding a Healthy Relationship with Food by Casey Crosbie and Wendy Sterling

Intuitive Eating, 4th Edition: A Revolutionary Anti-Diet Approach by Evelyn Tribole and Elyse Resch

The Intuitive Eating Workbook for Teens: A Non-Diet, Body Positive Approach to Building a Healthy Relationship with Food by Elyse Resch

Raising Body Positive Teens by Signe Darpinian, Wendy Sterling, and Shelley Aggarwal

Sick Enough: A Guide to the Medical Complications of Eating Disorders by Jennifer L. Gaudiani

Eating Disorder Websites

All the below eating disorder websites contain resources to help in finding treatment (provider directory/listings, helpline, and/or other referral service) as well as other information/resources related to eating disorders.

Academy for Eating Disorders (AED): www.aedweb.org

See Resources → Publications section for free downloads of *Eating Disorders: A Guide to Medical Care, 4th Edition* (3rd edition is available in multiple languages) and *Guidebook for Nutrition Treatment of Eating Disorders*. If you are unable to find providers who are eating disorder specialists, sharing these resources may be helpful to guide clinicians in caring for your dancer.

Beat Eating disorders: www.beateatingdisorders.org.uk

Butterfly Foundation: www.butterfly.org.au

Fighting Eating Disorders in Underrepresented Populations (FEDUP): www.fedupcollective.org

National Alliance for Eating Disorders: www.allianceforeatingdisorders.com and www.findedhelp.com

National Eating Disorders Collaboration (NEDC): www.nedc.com.au

National Eating Disorder Information Centre (NEDIC): www.nedic.ca

Project HEAL: www.theprojectheal.org

Screening and Assessment Tools

Female Athlete Triad: Screening Questions, Cumulative Risk Assessment tool, and Clearance and Return-to-Play Guidelines
Available at: https://doi.org/10.1136/bjsports-2013-093218

Male Athlete Triad: Screening Questions, Cumulative Risk Assessment tool, and Clearance and Return-to-Play Guidelines
Available at: https://doi.org/10.1097/jsm.0000000000000948

Relative Energy Deficiency in Sport Clinical Assessment Tool (RED-S CAT™)
Available at: https://bjsm.bmj.com/content/49/7/421

Safe Exercise at Every Stage Athlete (SEES-A) Guideline
Available at: https://www.safeexerciseateverystage.com/sees-guidelines

Eating Disorder Examination Questionnaire Short (EDE-QS)
Available at: https://doi.org/10.1371/journal.pone.0152744 (with additional information on scoring available at: https://doi.org/10.1186/s12888-020 -02565-5)

Eating Disorders Screen for Athletes (EDSA)
Available at: https://sites.google.com/view/edsa-screening-tool/home

Eating disorder Screen for Primary care (ESP)
Available at: https://www.ncbi.nlm.nih.gov/pmc/articles/PMC1494802/

InsideOut Institute Screener
Available at: https://insideoutinstitute.org.au/screener/

Other Websites

(*contains provider directory/listings)

Association for Size Diversity and Health* (ASDAH): www.asdah.org

AXIS Dance Company: www.axisdance.org

The Ellyn Satter Institute: www.ellynsatterinstitute.org

International Association for Dance Medicine & Science* (IADMS): www.iadms.org

MoBBallet (MoBB): www.mobballet.org

Moving For Equity Dancing Action: www.movingforequity.com

Self-Compassion, Dr. Kristin Neff: www.self-compassion.org

Sports and Human Performance Nutrition* (SHPN): www.shpndpg.org

Guidance for Finding Treatment Providers

Several of the websites listed in this Appendix provide directories of providers who work with eating disorders, dancers (i.e., IADMS), or athletes (i.e., SHPN). It's important to know that qualifications of the listed providers are not verified, and their training, experience, philosophy, and treatment approaches may vary greatly. I recommend asking the following questions to any treatment professional you are considering referring to or working with to ensure you find a qualified provider who best meets your needs:

What is your educational background, training, and experience in working with eating disorders and/or with dancers?
An eating disorder specialist needs the required credentials of their profession (e.g., Registered Dietitian [RD], Medical Doctor [MD], Licensed Clinical Social Worker [LCSW] or one of several other credentials for therapists) as well as additional training specifically in eating disorders. Look for providers with education, experience, and/or certifications/credentials that demonstrate expertise in working with clients with eating disorders.

It is also helpful if the provider has experience working with dancers. If you cannot find a provider with dance-specific experience, one who works with athletes may be a good fit (e.g., a dietitian specializing in sports nutrition). Asking the provider about the professional organizations they belong to and continuing education they have completed will provide additional insight into their training and experience (e.g., are they staying up to date with research and developments in eating disorder treatment?).

How many clients with eating disorders (and/or how many dancer clients) have you worked with?

An eating disorder provider should have several years of experience in the field and therefore have worked with numerous clients with eating disorders. Although it would be preferable to select a provider who has worked extensively with dancers, this may not always be possible. A qualified professional with an openness to learn more about dance-specific needs could still be a good fit.

What is your treatment philosophy and approach?

There are many different philosophies and approaches to providing nutritional, psychological, and medical care. Look for a provider who works in a way that feels like the best match for you. Regardless of their specific practice approach, I recommend finding professionals who provide evidence-based, trauma-informed, weight-inclusive care. When choosing a dietitian, I highly recommend working with one who uses a non-diet or intuitive eating approach.

Will you collaborate with other members of my treatment team?

The answer here should be yes. Particularly in eating disorder treatment, care collaboration is an essential component of providing good care.

Index

Page numbers in *italic* indicate a figure and page numbers in **bold** indicate a table on the corresponding page

For Product Safety Concerns and Information please contact our EU
representative GPSR@taylorandfrancis.com Taylor & Francis Verlag GmbH,
Kaufingerstraße 24, 80331 München, Germany

Printed and bound by CPI Group (UK) Ltd, Croydon, CR0 4YY

08/06/2025

01897008-0011